JIM I

MW00903301

DANA'S

A FATHER'S JOURNEY INTO

DISEASE

THE WORLD OF DIABETES

Dear Marc,
Thanks!

TRAFFORD

Canada • UK • USA • Spain

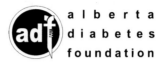

a l b e r t a
d i a b e t e s
f o u n d a t i o n

If you would like to support world leading diabetes research efforts at the
University of Alberta, home of the Edmonton Protocol, please contact:

Alberta Diabetes Foundation
12863—163 Street NW
Edmonton, Alberta, Canada, T5V 1K6

Phone: (780) 447 - 2643 • Email: info@afdr.ab.ca • Internet: www.afdr.ab.ca

PROCEEDS FROM THE SALE OF THIS BOOK WILL BE DONATED TO SUPPORT DIABETES RESEARCH

Note for Librarians: a cataloguing record for this book that includes Dewey Decimal Classification and US Library of
Congress numbers is available from the Library and Archives of Canada. The complete cataloguing record can be obtained
from their online database at: www.collectionscanada.ca/amicus/index-e.html

ISBN 1-4120-4347-6

Printed in Victoria, BC, Canada

TRAFFORD

Offices in Canada, USA, Ireland, UK and Spain

This book was published *on-demand* in cooperation with Trafford Publishing. On-demand publishing is a unique process and
service of making a book available for retail sale to the public taking advantage of on-demand manufacturing and Internet
marketing. On-demand publishing includes promotions, retail sales, manufacturing, order fulfilment, accounting and collecting
royalties on behalf of the author.

Book sales for North America and international:

Trafford Publishing, 6E–2333 Government St., Victoria, BC v8t 4p4 CANADA

phone 250 383 6864 (toll-free 1 888 232 4444) • fax 250 383 6804; email to orders@trafford.com

Book sales in Europe:

Trafford Publishing (uk) Ltd., Enterprise House, Wistaston Road Business Centre,

Wistaston Road, Crewe, Cheshire cw2 7rp UNITED KINGDOM

phone 01270 251 396 (local rate 0845 230 9601) • facsimile 01270 254 983; orders.uk@trafford.com

Order online at:

www.trafford.com/robots/04-2155.html

10 9 8 7 6 5 4 3

"I have spent my career trying to stop diabetes with science. Jim Kanerva delivers a heartfelt and realistic account of the human impact of this insidious disease. Dana's Disease helps to illuminate why I continue my work."

—Ray Rajotte, PhD

PROFESSOR OF SURGERY AND MEDICINE
FOUNDER AND DIRECTOR OF ISLET TRANSPLANT GROUP
DIRECTOR OF THE SURGICAL-MEDICAL RESEARCH INSTITUTE
SCIENTIFIC DIRECTOR OF THE ALBERTA DIABETES INSTITUTE
ALBERTA DIABETES FOUNDATION DIRECTOR

For Dana, Ross, and Eric
So that you know you are loved
and that Mom and Dad will be there

TERMS TO KNOW FOR THIS BOOK

Acceptable Pre-meal Blood Sugar Level: 5.0–7.2 mmol/l
(90–130 mg/dl)

Acceptable Post-meal Blood Sugar Level: Less than 10.0 mmol/l
(180 mg/dl)

1 mmol/l = 18 mg/dl

1 unit of insulin in Dana's ultra fine needles =   1/100 cc or 1/100 ml
100 units of insulin in Dana's ultra fine needles =   1 cc or 1 ml

Acknowledgements

This project could not have moved forward if it were not for the love and support of my family. Writing this book was a personal journey of discovery, healing, and moving forward for me. For the development of this book and for the commitment shown to me I am truly grateful—

—to my wife Laurie, who provided endless support and valuable input throughout the writing and editing process, not to mention the extra work around the house she did to cover for me while I wrote.

—to my sister Raili, who spent considerable time editing my work for style and content, which was no easy task.

—to Ray, Judy, Norm, Marg, Christine, Scotty, Maureen, Dave, Bill, Kim, Al, Susan, Craig, Steve, Marilyn, and Rob for taking the time to read the book and provide constructive feedback.

—to Dr. Ray Rajotte and his wife Gloria for taking the time to read this book, provide constructive feedback, and for endorsing it.

—to Don Oborowsky, Ted Degner, Terry Devine, and Dave Muir for their generous support.

Contents

CHAPTER 1

Day 1:
Wednesday November 13, 2002

It was about 4:25 pm, five minutes to the end of the workday. The phone rang, distracting me in the middle of writing a disciplinary letter to a chronically absent welder.

"Jim?" my wife Laurie demanded before I got the receiver to my ear.

"Hi."

"Can you stop by the grocery store on your way home and pick up some Canada Dry Ginger Ale? Dana needs some."

I diverted my thoughts away from work, trying to get in tune with Laurie's problem. "Does it have to be diet?"

"Why would she need diet? She's not keeping anything down. Her flu's getting worse. She needs the extra carbs."

"Take a breath man! Do you want me to flatten it before I get home too?"

"Don't be an ass. Are you going to get the ginger ale or

not?" she snapped.

"Yes, I'm going to get it."

There was silence and then a sigh. "I love you," Laurie offered. "I'm sorry, I'm just tense."

"I love you too but I don't understand this Laurie. We all got the flu shot. How can she have the flu?"

"The flu shot only protects you against the three major strains for this flu season. It doesn't protect you against them all," Laurie explained.

I pressed her further. "When we had the nurses come in and give out flu shots at work, I'm sure they said that the shot would also make the symptoms of the flu much less severe if you did get it. Dana's symptoms are getting worse."

"I don't know where those people got their information, but I've never heard that. I'll ask Dad and Al, but Dad didn't mention that to me when he gave Eric, Ross, Dana, and I the shot a few weeks ago."

"Do you think Dad and Al know what the hell they're talking about in this case?"

"They're doctors, Jim! What do you think, they're making it up?"

"Fine!" I answered, leaning back in my chair, looking at the ceiling now. "I'm leaving work right now and I'll pick up the pop for Dana. Do you need anything else?"

"Yes, I almost forgot. Can you pick up a few packs of Lifesavers and some real juice Popsicles?"

"No problem," I sighed. "I'll see you in a few minutes."

At 4:30 pm, I said good night to a few employees and left Waiward Steel Fabricators, the structural steel fabrication plant where I work. I drove my used white SUV home, south on 34th street through the rich industrial area and east into the bedroom community of Sherwood Park on the clogged freeway. I stopped in at the Nottingham IGA, picked up Laurie's groceries, then quickly popped into the Blockbuster Video and rented a movie. If everybody went to bed early tonight, as I expected, I'd need the movie to entertain myself later. My watch showed the time as 4:50 pm. I quickened my pace a little in case Dana needed any of the groceries for her supper at 5:00 pm. I arrived at our new home just a few minutes before 5:00 pm.

Supper was always at 5:00 pm. Laurie allowed it to be as late as 5:30 pm for special occasions from time to time, but not too often. The reason for this strict routine was Dana, my nearly-six-year-old Type 1 diabetic daughter. Food is medicine for a Type 1 diabetic. Our sons, four-year-old Ross and 16-month-old Eric were healthy, thank God.

When I walked in the house the usual mob of greetings and hugs from kids and our black lab-cross Sasha met me at the garage door. Dana was lying on the couch and didn't move. Her hug was usually first. She just stared at the TV with an expressionless face. Dana was a fair skinned, blonde child to begin with. She was short and only weighed about 40 pounds, but at her best was pretty, athletic, and smart. However, now Dana looked gaunt, pale, and lifeless.

"Has she eaten anything today?" I asked, sitting down to a plate of rice, vegetables, and chicken.

"No," Laurie replied. "Why do you think I asked for the ginger ale?"

I took a few bites of food, got up from the table and made my way over to Dana. "Aren't you going to come and try to eat some supper, Dana?" I begged her in a whisper.

"I'm not hungry, Daddy."

I picked her up to give her a hug and her left ear banged against my chest.

"Ow! Ow! That hurts! Put me down. Put me down now, Daddy!" Dana screamed and hit me with her fists with much more force than I thought she would be capable of in her weakened state.

I laid her roughly back on the couch and looked at her with some anger.

"Jim. Remember she has an ear infection right now. Don't bang her around and wrestle," Laurie scolded.

"I didn't hit her ear. It just touched my chest as I picked her up."

Laurie continued, "Leave her alone and come eat some supper. I'll feed her something in a few minutes."

"What was her blood sugar when you checked it before supper?" I asked.

"Four point six."

I was not highly involved in the daily management of Dana's disease, and was curious about how this should be handled. "Are you giving her any insulin tonight?"

"No quick-acting for sure, but I might give her one unit of long-acting," she replied.

I finished my dinner and Laurie unwrapped one of the Popsicles. Dana needed 36 grams of carbohydrates for dinner. That wasn't going to happen tonight. If she ate her full meal, she would get 2.5 units of long-acting insulin and 0.5 units of quick-acting. If her blood sugar was above 15 mmol/litre we'd give an extra 0.5 units of quick-acting to bring it back down to the target of between 5 to 10 mmol/l. When Dana was sick, you had to manage her eating, blood sugar, mood, and insulin as best you could. Any control we had was at best fleeting and at worst removed. Being sick did weird and inexplicable things to Dana's blood sugar. She could eat nothing and be high or eat like a ravenous animal and be low. Nothing made sense, so we increased the number of times we'd check her blood sugar from five times per day to, in this case, hourly at least.

It was a sobering feeling entering an evening like this. As the darkness of night took over, it felt as though we were preparing for a battle. I knew that Laurie and I would have to manage Dana's condition all night. If her blood sugar dropped below 3.5 mmol/l, we'd have lost the fight and would be forced to retreat and bring her in for an intravenous treatment at the University of Alberta Hospital to stabilize her.

Laurie started to clean the supper dishes. I walked over to the couch that Dana had chosen to rest on in our great room, sat down beside her and offered her the orange Popsicle. She sat up, took it from me, and began to suck on it. "Thank you, Daddy."

"You're welcome, Dana-Banayna. What are you watching?"

"Sponge Bob."

"Sponge Bob! Of course, how could Daddy not have known that you'd be watching that most educational of shows?"

Dana just stared at me, not sure what to make of the sarcasm. Rossco and Eric finished their supper and bounded into the great room to watch. We watched TV and I wrestled with the boys a little so they could burn off some energy. Snack time, 7:30 pm, snuck up quickly. The boys fought for a seat at the table then wolfed down half a banana and a cookie each. Dana's blood sugar was still uncomfortably low. She hadn't eaten enough carbohydrates at supper and she needed 25 grams more at bedtime snack. She came to the table and forced down some of the ginger ale and a piece of white bread.

"What are you doing?" Laurie demanded. "She's throwing up the bread, Jim. I tried toast this morning."

"She hasn't thrown up since I've been home," I reasoned. "Did you ever think maybe the worst has passed? Besides, bread will help to sponge up the gurgling of all that acid down in her stomach."

"It won't work!" Laurie responded, warning me more sternly.

Dana slowly finished the pop and bread and went back to the couch to lie down. Laurie took Rossco and Eric upstairs to brush their teeth, read two stories, and go to bed. I made myself a frozen blueberry and apple juice slushy and sat down with Dana again.

"Can Daddy watch his movie now, while you try to go to sleep?"

"Can I stay on the couch?" Dana asked.

"Yes, you can stay down here."

"Okay, Daddy."

She cuddled in tight to my stomach and chest with her back to me, as I lay sideways on the couch watching the movie. We remained in that position for the better part of 20 minutes when Dana began to whine and complain about her stomach. "I don't feel well, Daddy. I'm going to throw up."

"Don't wait here, honey. Get up! Go to the bathroom!" I ordered Dana.

Dana got up from the couch cradling her stomach and dashed to the main floor bathroom with me scrambling behind her. She didn't quite reach the toilet bowl before she started some torturous retching. Once she'd finished, there was vomit on the walls and the floor of the bathroom, as well as in the toilet.

"I told you the bread wouldn't work," Laurie complained, coming down the stairs.

"It hurts, Daddy. It hurts my throat," Dana cried as she wiped her mouth with the arm of her pajamas and leaned weakly against me.

I knelt on the bathroom floor beside her, both of us waiting for the next retch.

"I know it hurts, Dana," I reassured her in a strong voice. "Daddy's had the flu many times and I've had to throw up, too. You just have to do it and get it over with."

Dana's stomach muscles tightened once more and she dipped her head into the toilet bowl again. She heaved and vomited, only expelling bile by this point, and cried out for Mommy between the forceful thrusts of her stomach. When she knew it was done she rested her head on the cool toilet seat and wept.

I carried her upstairs where Laurie met us with clean pajamas and a warm face cloth to clean Dana.

"Do you want to go to sleep in your own bed for a while,

Dana?" Laurie asked.

"No, Mommy, I'm scared. Can I please stay downstairs with you and Daddy?"

Laurie looked at me, searching for my take on the situation. Situations like these came up for us all the time with the kids, where we would get stumped on the smallest decision amidst whatever else might be going on at the time. It was easy for us to get lost micromanaging some situation, allowing the bigger issue to grow unchecked.

"I don't care, I guess. She should go to bed, but if you're okay with it, fine."

"Fine, Dana. You can lay down on the couch with Daddy," Laurie soothed.

Before Laurie walked away, I asked: "Do you want me to do her blood sugar again, Lo?"

"Yes, please, I forgot. It's been more than an hour for sure by now."

Dana went back to the couch and handed me her right arm. I picked my favourite spot to poke her with the well-used lancet. We were supposed to change the lancet each time we completed a blood sugar test. When she was first diagnosed, Laurie and I were both religious about this. Now, it was a pain in the ass, so we left the lancet in until we had the motivation to change it, sometimes for weeks. My favourite spot to poke Dana was on her right thumb, on a tender spot of the flesh. This was just underneath the left side of her thumbnail, about a quarter of an inch toward the middle of the meat. I tried my best to rotate finger poke locations to avoid callusing, but was often drawn to this same spot. I poked her thumb and squeezed it for blood. Dana had been poked so many times she didn't even pay attention anymore.

"What is it?" Laurie asked from the kitchen, looking up from her Edmonton Journal crossword puzzle.

"It's only four point two," I answered, disappointed.

"She did just throw up."

"We still have to get it up over seven somehow to get any real sleep tonight," I responded, rubbing my eyes.

Laurie looked down at the words on her crossword for a moment and then suggested, "Try another Popsicle."

"No, Mommy!" Dana whined. "I don't want anything else to eat. No more, please."

"Dana. You have to keep eating or we have to go to the hospital to get an IV. You know that," Laurie explained.

I sat on the couch with my back leaning against the arm and my legs stretched out lengthwise across the couch. Dana climbed into my lap and covered herself with her blanket, pulling it tight to her chin. Laurie brought her another Popsicle and handed it to me. I unwrapped it and offered it to Dana. She reluctantly agreed, slowly licking at the real strawberry treat. We watched the movie for less than half an hour more when Dana's teeth began to chatter and her legs began to shake.

"What's the problem Dana?" I asked, becoming slightly frustrated with the progression of this flu.

"It hurts, Daddy."

"What hurts, Dana?"

"My head and my stomach," She responded, continuing to make an irritating whine between her chattering teeth.

"She's got a fever you know," I said, looking over at Laurie.

"Yes, I know, Jim," Laurie replied.

"Dana, you're going to have to tough this out a little bit. It's only the flu. I know it hurts, but you're going to be fine," I lectured her in a calm, but firm voice. "Suck it up a little bit and try not to complain about the pain so much."

"She's still taking antibiotics for her ear infection," Laurie informed me. "I think her ear is bothering her too."

"I can tell her ear is bothering her, Laurie. I just don't think she has to whine so much."

Laurie and I continued the blood sugar testing and feeding attempts until the movie was over and midnight had slipped by. Dana hadn't vomited for a couple of hours so we decided to put her into her own bed.

"Where's Sasha? I need Sasha!" Dana pleaded as I covered her with her Barbie comforter in her canopy bed.

Dana always slept with Sasha. She and the dog had a special bond. It had been Sasha's job to protect Dana while she was going to sleep since Dana first saw the White Face in her closet at the old house and screamed out in the middle of the night.

I called the dog to her room. Sasha jumped on Dana's bed and lay down at the end, leaving Dana enough room to stretch out. Then Laurie and I readied for bed and the long night ahead. "How's the dog today? Did she eat anything?" I asked.

"No. I don't know, maybe the vet's right. Do you think we should do the exploratory surgery?" Laurie asked.

"Not a chance! That surgery is expensive. Sasha will be nine years old in a few months. That's already pretty old for a

Lab. If they do the surgery and find cancer, they can't stop it. If they don't find cancer we wasted the money. What's the point of the surgery? Let's keep trying the ulcer medication first."

Laurie thought for a moment. "I guess that's fine. I'll keep feeding her the ulcer medication. She's dropping fur all over the house like crazy. She's just not well. If she died at least I wouldn't have to vacuum."

"Stop that!"

"I'm only kidding," Laurie shot back.

Laurie continued to do her crossword puzzle and I rolled over to go to sleep. She would manage the night. If she needed me to get up with Dana, she'd let me know.

"Set your alarm for 1:30 am," Laurie ordered.

I set the alarm and closed my eyes. I thought of Father Wes. Without speaking, I said a prayer. I asked God, whatever that was, to keep Laurie safe and to give her endurance through Dana's flu. I asked God to keep Dana, Ross, and Eric safe and healthy. I asked God to heal Sasha so that she could be with us for a few more years. I thanked God for our home and my job. I asked that my anger and disillusionment with God and religions be forgiven.

I wondered if saying any of that would help at all. Then I drifted off to sleep.

CHAPTER 2

Sunday January 16, 2000

It was still dark out, but I could see a light snow falling on our 30-year old Sherwood Park bungalow. I felt a slight draft coming from the tiny hole in the drywall behind the baseboard in the corner, behind where the laundry basket sat. "We need a new house," I thought.

The clock read 6:22 am. Laurie was still sleeping, but I could hear from across the hall that Dana was up early, as usual. Fourteen-month old Rossco was still in his crib and was not much of an early riser. He preferred to sleep until 9:00 am or later, if we'd let him. Not Dana. She had too much energy and wanted to do too many things. She turned a precocious three on January 2.

I laid back and remembered the great party that we had at my parent's home on New Year's Eve this past year. It was a blowout for a special New Year's Day, January 1, 2000. It wasn't a bar-party like I used to attend in university. I was past that stage. We had a five-course fondue, with each family responsible to bring a different course and wine. At midnight, my sister Susan and her husband Craig brought out the 1990 Dom Perrignon they'd bought in the summer. We toasted to all of the good fortune that we had: great kids, good jobs, good health, and good homes. Overall, it was a joyful Christmas season, complete with Christmas Eve with my family at my parent's home and Christmas Day with Laurie's family at her mom and dad's.

Dana snuck into our room, looking to see if we were awake. She crept quietly to my side of the bed, and I helped the game along by pretending to be asleep.

"Daddy? Dad? Are you up?"

I lay motionless until Dana gently poked my face.

"Daddy? Are you up?"

"Huh? What, what?"

I slowly opened my eyes just in time to spasm and gag as Sasha gave me a slobbery kiss right on my lips. Dana laughed, covering her mouth trying to be quiet.

"Daddy. Hungry. Cook breakfast. Please?"

I rolled my eyes and looked at her again. "Now?"

"Yes."

I completed our almost ritualistic Sunday procession. First, I stretched while lying in bed, making a roaring lion sound, and then picked her up and held her aloft by her tummy. She held onto the window ledge, kept her legs together and parallel to the bed, and could just see out of the window. "What do you see, Dana?"

"The garage. Big tree."

"The big Christmas tree in the back yard?"

"Yes."

"What else?"

"I'm hungry, Daddy."

I eased her back down onto my chest and gave her a hug. I loved Dana's hugs. They were to die for. Dana had pretty much been a Mommy's girl for a long time. She wouldn't let me hold her much when she was smaller and not at all if she was hurt or scared. Then Ross was born. That changed everything in the relationship. Suddenly, Dana was second fiddle. Ross had Mom's attention, of which he demanded the lion's share. Dana found herself short on quite a bit of Mommy face-time. That's where I came in. I may be second choice to Mommy, but at least my daughter now wanted to be near me and do some Daddy things. When she hugged me I picked her up, she buried her face under my chin, wrapped her arms tightly around my neck, and closed her eyes. "What do you want, Dana-Banayna? You can eat anything you want."

"French toast?" she said, clapping her hands.

"With lots of cinnamon and maple syrup?" I asked.

"Yes!"

"Okay."

Dana and I left Mom and Rossco sleeping and went into our small kitchen. She sat at the table and waited while I poured her a big glass of apple juice and peeled an orange.

We didn't have a flat-bottomed bowl to mix the batter that was big enough to fit a slice of bread, so I used the spare frying pan. I measured out the mixture of eggs, milk, sugar, cinnamon, and vanilla.

We'd had some guests over for dinner the night before,

which meant there was some one-day old San Francisco sourdough bread in the fridge, and that I had a slight hangover. I cut a thick slice of the beautiful bread and laid it in the three-egg mixture, allowing the bread to soak up lots of batter through multiple flips. Then I placed it in the hot pan with melted margarine. Within minutes Dana had a hot slice of French toast on her plate to go with everything else. "Do you want real maple syrup on that, Dana, or jam?"

"Oh yeah, maple syrup!"

She gobbled about half of it before slowing her pace because she was feeling full. I made a small batch of flavoured scrambled eggs out of the remainder of the batter and toasted some bread for myself while Dana was eating. In short order I'd eaten my food as well.

"Do you want to watch a Daddy movie with me?" I asked.

"Yes! Daddy movie! Ice Planet! Ice Planet!"

I had always been a huge Star Wars fan. I was seven years old, and was immediately smitten for life when the first Star Wars movie was released in theatres. It was fun to share my love of Star Wars with Dana. The two of us went downstairs and put in *The Empire Strikes Back*. The basement was cold as it lacked a floor heating vent, and the fireplace, while not lit, allowed a river of winter air to flow into the room, covering the carpet with a thick frosty layer. I started a fire and cuddled under a polar fleece blanket on the couch with Dana as the movie started.

About half-way through, Laurie came downstairs and said good morning. "Do you guys want to come to church with Ross and I?"

"Yes, Mommy!" Dana yelled.

"Thanks, honey! You just killed my party," I scowled.

"You could come with us too, you know. It might do you some good."

"I'm not going to church. I've got a thousand better things to do with my time than go there."

"Jim, you don't have to be so harsh about it."

"Come on Laurie, I don't have to visit a glorified social club to get close to God, or whatever, or to be a good person. I would rather concentrate on being good for the whole week than on making sure that I go to church for one hour on Sunday."

"I don't agree with you. I wish you'd just come. It would be good for the kids, you know."

"You go."

Laurie shook her head in disgust and took Dana up to her room to get her ready. Soon they were gone. I stopped the movie that I'd seen dozens of times and went upstairs to read the Sunday Edmonton Journal. The mail from the week was still unopened on the baker's stand. I leafed through it and put the bills to the side. The banking and bill paying was Laurie's job. It was a waste of my time to read through banking information or bills, as Laurie could not relinquish any control of that job and retain her sanity.

I placed the copy of Sports Illustrated under the paper and would read through the magazine after going through the paper. There were also two letters from charities. One was from the Canadian Diabetes Association and one was from the Canadian Liver Foundation. I opened the letters and quickly scanned them. Having appeased my conscience by reading their requests for donations, I tossed the letters in the garbage. With that, I went back to reading the paper.

Laurie and the kids arrived home shortly after noon. "Daddy, brunch?" Dana yelled.

"Okay, okay," I agreed.

I picked myself off the chair and dressed in some track pants and a comfortable rugby shirt. Laurie had already loaded the kids in the green minivan.

"I thought that we were going for brunch, Lo?" I asked, folding my arms, as we pulled into the Dairy Queen parking lot.

"It was Dana's choice. She wants a Blizzard with Smarties in it. What could I say? Besides, you're not dressed for much more than Dairy Queen."

"Thanks," I retorted.

The burgers, fries, and pop came quickly, and Dana was digging into her Blizzard in no time.

"Can you do something with the kids and me this afternoon, Jim?" Laurie asked with a soft smile.

"I was going to go into work to finish a little paperwork this afternoon."

"It's Sunday, and Dana wants to do something with you. Rossco could burn some energy off too. Can't you skip work this weekend?"

I stared off across Baseline Road watching the cars drive by, rubbing my forehead with my hand.

"Jim? Jim, please answer?"

"Yeah, okay," I answered. "I looked through the mail this

morning. We got letters from diabetes and liver charities. You didn't want to give anything did you?"

"We haven't given that much this year. Did you want to give?"

"I threw them out."

Laurie shrugged her shoulders and continued to gather up all of the trash onto one of the lunch trays.

"What do you want to do with the kids, Jim?"

"I suppose we could go swimming this afternoon. Dana and I haven't been going on our regular Thursday swim since the Christmas season started."

Dana clapped her hands and beamed. Rossco did too, although I'm certain that he had no idea what the hell was going on.

"Oh, by the way, my mom called and invited us to dinner tonight. Do you want to go?" Laurie asked.

I thought about it for a few seconds as I dumped the remnants of our lunch into the trash and placed the tray back on top of the garbage can.

"I suppose so. When does she want us there?"

"Five-ish."

We loaded our family into the minivan and darted home just long enough to pick up the swimming bags and be on our way again. "Which pool are we going to?" I inquired.

"Blue pool!" Dana yelled, referring to the Sherwood Park Kinsmen Pool with the deep blue dive tank.

"Fine. The blue pool it is."

When we arrived at the pool Laurie took Rossco into the girls' change room and I took Dana into the boys'. Dana and I changed quickly, showered, and headed for the pool deck. She looked up at me, grabbed my hand, and pulled me hard to the right.

"Big slide?"

I nodded and burst up the dripping rusted spiral staircase toward the indoor two-storey waterslide. Dana scrambled up the ladder and turned to wait for me.

"Daddy's first," I ordered.

Dana nodded and moved to the side. I waited until the light turned green as the previous slider hit the foaming water below. "Remember Dana, wait until it's green before you go. Okay?"

"Okay, Daddy."

I slipped down the two sloping and dropping twists of the waterslide and plunged into the water, holding my glasses so they didn't fall off my balding head. I stopped in the middle of the high-current, foaming water about ten feet from the exit lip of the slide and waited for Dana. In seconds she was coming around the last corner on her knees, laughing, with her hands raised. She completed a 360 degree turn and plunged into the water, disappearing below the surface.

The teenage lifeguard exploded from his chair to the edge of the pool scanning the water for Dana, the swimmer in distress.

"She's okay," I reassured the concerned boy. "She can swim like a fish."

A split second later, Dana resurfaced on her back, spitting a stream of water toward the ceiling. Just before her head would have banged the tile edge of the pool deck she flipped and grabbed the edge with her hands. "That was fun, Daddy! Can we go to the blue pool now?"

I surveyed the scene for a few seconds to find Laurie and Ross. She waved at me from the kiddy pool.

"Do you want to go play with Rossco and Mommy in the kiddy pool first?"

"No. Blue pool."

"Say please, Dana."

"Please. Blue pool."

"Alright, let's go."

Dana skipped to the 1.5 metre diving board, which did not have any kids waiting on it. She climbed up the ladder and walked with purpose to the end of the board. Dana was so small that she looked no more than two. She wiped her blonde hair away from her face, fixed her big one piece Barbie swimsuit that gaped on her tiny little body, and gave me a wide grin as I jumped into the pool. I swam out to about five feet in front of the diving board. Without any hesitation, she put her hands together, lined her feet up together, fell forward, and completed a decent head-first dive. She paused under the water for a few seconds, spun around while vertical, and then broke the surface.

The feat had caught the attention of another lifeguard and she quickly walked over to the edge of the pool to meet Dana and me as we exited.

"You can't be in the water with her if she is going to use the diving board. She has to be able to do it all by herself."

"That's fine," I smirked with pride. "Dana, can you do it all by yourself?"

"Yes!"

With that she walked back over to the diving board, climbed up the ladder, walked to the end, and repeated the dive once more. The lifeguard mumbled something and was on her way. Another male lifeguard walked over to me. "She has to be able to swim a length of the dive tank by herself if she's going to be in here without a life jacket."

"What? We've been swimming at this pool for two years and I've never heard that rule."

"I can't imagine why. It's always been a rule in Strathcona County."

"Come on you guys," I laughed. "She can swim. She's been swimming in front of you guys like this for six months already."

"She does the length or you put her in a life jacket."

"I hear you. Dana, can you jump in and swim across the pool beside the floating rope?"

She nodded, jumped in, and started across the pool doing a mock-frog kind of stroke. A few feet from the edge she took a gulp of air, pulled hard with her arms, and coasted to the edge of the pool with her head below the surface. Dana pulled herself out of the water and we walked back toward the diving board. In the meantime, the young lifeguard had closed it. He had won. I could only laugh and rub Dana's head admiringly as she hugged my leg, not understanding what had just taken place.

We swam a little bit more with Rossco and Laurie and then made our way home. It was time to pack up and head into St. Albert to Laurie's parent's house for dinner. The minivan had grooved that road many times over the last month during the holiday season. Soon we were all seated at the table at Laurie's parents, Norm and Marg, while they served their children and grandchildren dinner.

The family was close knit, Catholic, feisty, and smart. Laurie had two older sisters, one younger sister, and one younger brother. Norm and Marg were generous, helpful, and pushed for the best in all around them by leading by example. All of Laurie's siblings were married and had children. In fact, there were already nine grandchildren in the family by this point and all were seated at the kid's table. The twelve adults sat at the dining room table. My mouth watered as our hosts served one of my favourite winter meals, roast beef, roasted potatoes, carrots, and Yorkshire pudding with gravy.

The conversation at these dinners was usually stimulating and intelligent, but too often became voracious, like a shark's feeding frenzy. The constant din from the kid's table set the mood perfectly on edge for another good debate. The event would always start out with the requisite small talk such as inquiring about work, current events, and politics. The food was eaten and the wine flowed mostly into the men. Eventually, the conversation would meander and the predators would attack.

"So did the millennium bug shut down the computers at everyone's offices?" Laurie's younger sister Kim inquired with mock concern.

"What a crock that whole thing was," Kim's husband Bill added.

"Oh God," I jumped in. "Our company bought into that hysteria all the way. All any of us know is that there were no problems on January first or second. But the computer industry would have us believe that they prevented that."

"I'd like to know how many consultants stole money from companies during that hoax?" my older brother-in-law Scotty piped up.

"There's the teacher complaining again about somebody else making more money than him," Bill observed with a smile, knowing he'd inflicted the first wound.

Laurie's oldest sister Christine quickly came to her husband's defense. "Scotty wouldn't be complaining about his salary if an entire province of morons like Bill and Jim didn't continue to vote for our idiot premier."

"What should we do, vote for your Liberal candidate?" I waded in. "What's her name, Nancy MacBeth the Liberal or is it what she once was, Nancy Betkowski the jaded conservative that lost to Klein?"

"Can we be excused?" Christine's oldest daughter Julia asked, as the ambassador for all of the kids.

"Yes," Scotty answered, resulting in a mass exodus of children to the basement to watch TV and play dress up.

"You'd better add me to that list of Klein voters," Laurie quietly added.

"Christine, you just can't handle being at the table with two Alberta red necks like Jimmy and I," Bill stated, after sarcastically sniffing, rubbing his nose and putting his arm around me.

"You two are ridiculous," Christine returned. "Who'd have guessed that Jim the engineer and Bill the business owner would vote like that? Only lawyers should be allowed to vote because we're the only group that knows what the hell is going on in politics."

"Can we stop this and talk about something else?" Kim begged.

"Dana and Ross were good at church today," Laurie offered, hoping to change the subject to something friendlier.

"Liam and Mackenzie were also good," Kim stated. "Bill came to church today too."

"Did Jim go to church with you today?" Marg asked, looking at Laurie.

"No," Laurie reluctantly answered.

Marg had been patiently paying attention to the topics of conversation taking place and had now found one close to one of her interests. She had been making a strong effort to bring God closer to her in her life and to try to understand her faith.

"Why don't you go to church, Jim?" Marg inquired.

"Why is it so important to go?" I responded, sensing that I was the only target at the table now.

"To bring God closer to you," Laurie's brother Al answered after being unusually quiet.

"You don't need to be in the building to be close to God," I added.

"Yes, but it helps," Marg contributed.

"Helps with what?" I asked.

"It helps you to know God and to have him be in your life," Laurie explained.

"Oh boy, here we go again," Christine sighed.

"What was that about?" Laurie asked defensively.

"I don't believe in the existence of an interfering spirit,"

Christine explained. "I just can't see that being true."

"I disagree," Laurie argued. "I feel God close to me when I pray, like we're having a conversation. I can see his work in my daily life and I believe that he impacts my life directly. Some of my prayers have been answered."

"Come on. Are you trying to tell us that God speaks to you directly?" Christine asked, pointing at Laurie. "Are you saying that he answers your prayers because you asked him to? Give me a break! Millions of people around the world suffer horrible atrocities every day and many die horrible deaths. There are significant problems on this planet that go unsolved. Do you really expect me to believe that your little prayers are actually answered?"

"I have to agree with Christine," I interjected. "I can't believe that God, if he truly were an interfering spirit, would ignore such significant problems to answer what are, in comparison, insignificant issues like ours."

Laurie was beginning to get angry. "You guys can't just dismiss the results of my faith because you don't believe, and furthermore-"

"Who wants coffee or tea?" Kim and Marg interrupted.

"Are you guys implying that I am lying about my relationship with God?" Laurie asked, ignoring Marg and Kim.

"No. We're just saying what you're suggesting is ridiculous," Christine answered.

"This is such bull! I don't have to listen to this crap!" Laurie yelled as she pushed back from the table and left the room.

"I'll take that to mean you don't want any tea then Laurie?" Marg mumbled as Laurie left the room.

"Mom!" Laurie retorted.

Bill poured me another glass of wine and one for himself. We drank a couple of sips during the long quiet aftermath of the verbal jousting match. Finally, after finishing his glass, he looked around the table, cleared his throat, threw his hands in the air, and in a loud and obnoxious voice announced: "I win again!"

Al looked at Bill, looked away, and started to laugh. "Bill, you're such an ass."

CHAPTER 3

Saturday May 27, 2000

"Dana?" I whispered quietly into my daughter's ear as I shook her head against her pillow. "Dana, wake up. Dana, wake up. It's a beautiful day."

I gave up trying for the moment and returned to the kitchen table in our old house to sit with Laurie and Ross. The sun was up, the possibilities for the day were endless and my energetic three-year-old daughter was still sleeping.

"What do you think is wrong with her?" Laurie asked.

"I don't know. She's growing. That takes a lot of energy, you know," I answered assertively, trying my best to ease Laurie's concern.

"I'm worried. Julia has been having all of these urinary tract problems. Christine and Scotty have been taking her to specialists for years and they still haven't solved all of the infection issues. I don't even think the doctors know what is causing the problem."

"You don't think that Dana has an infection there do you?"

"I took her to see Al a few weeks ago. Remember? They did some blood work on her. It came up negative."

"That's good. Isn't it?"

"Yes, but what's the problem?"

"I told you. She's just getting bigger and it's using up a lot of her energy. She's not a big kid. It'll get better. You'll see."

Laurie smiled at my attempt to reassure her again, leaned over, and we kissed. Then she pushed back from the table, got up, and went into Dana's room. Within minutes Dana was up and walking toward the kitchen. Her eyes were only partially open and she was rubbing them vigorously, whining a little about being woken so early. She was walking like an old drunk, or maybe like me drunk, which made me laugh. Ross was oblivious to the entire scene as he continued to eat his toast and jam and sliced apples. His face was covered with jam and margarine and he wasn't wasting any energy on talking at all.

Dana finally sat down at the table as Laurie was clearing the dishes. I made a plate of toast and sliced fruit for Dana and served her.

"Can I have juice?" she asked. "I'm thirsty."

"Sure," Laurie answered, pouring her a big glass of orange juice.

The phone rang. Laurie answered. She moved into the living room behind the kitchen wall to get some privacy as Ross, Dana, and I worked at having a conversation. Within a few minutes, Laurie returned. "Your mom is inviting everybody over today for dinner. Do you want to go?"

"Sure," I answered. "Hey kids, do you want to go to Grammy and Papa's tonight?"

"Yes! Grammy's!" Dana answered, clapping her hands and smiling.

Ross looked up from his plate, with his mouth full of food, and nodded his head, complete with his considerable baby-double chin.

"I was actually hoping to go my parents' for a swim in the pool and dinner today, Jim. Do you really want to go to your mom's?"

"Laurie. We go to your parents' and visit your family often. My family doesn't visit as often. I want to go to my mom's tonight."

Laurie appeared a little disappointed, but agreed. "Can we at least go over to my mom's for a swim before going for dinner?"

"Alright," I responded. "When do you want to go?"

"Why don't we get there for early afternoon? Then I can put Rossco down for a nap and Dana, you, and I can go swimming."

Dana and Ross finished their breakfast and went downstairs to watch some TV. Laurie and I packed our swim bag and a few bottles of wine from the basement for dinner. By a little after noon we were in the minivan driving to Norm and Marg's house in St. Albert.

When we arrived, I looked back to see that Ross and Dana had fallen asleep during the ride over. We knew this drill too well. As carefully and as quietly as possible I unbuckled Ross and lifted his 30 pound, 19 month-old bulk, rested his head on my left shoulder and carried him upstairs. I whispered hello while passing Marg, who was holding the front door open for us. Laurie gently shook Dana in her car seat to wake her from her short nap so that she could get up and go for a swim.

"Wake up, Dana. Come on honey, we're at Grandma's. It's time for swimming!"

"Leave me alone," Dana whined as she pushed Laurie's hands away and started to cry.

"Come on Dana, let's get up and go swimming. Come on! Swimming is your favourite."

"Go away!" Dana screamed as she finally opened her eyes and pounded her seat in protest to being stirred from her sleep.

Laurie became disgusted with Dana's rudeness, unbuckled her, and dragged her out of the car kicking and crying.

"Here. Take her. I've heard enough of this," Laurie growled as she handed Dana off to me on the driveway and went inside to sit down and talk with Marg.

"What's wrong, Dana?" I asked in a soothing voice as she buried her head into the side of my neck and continued to cry.

"I'm tired," she sobbed.

"Don't you want to go swimming with Daddy?"

"No. Sleep."

"Dana Banayna, I've been waiting all morning to go swimming with you. Won't you come with me? It's my favourite thing to do with you."

Dana sobbed for a few more seconds, pulled her head back from my neck, and loosened her hug grip. "Alright, Daddy."

"That's my girl."

I put her down on my right side and extended my hand down to her. She put her left hand out, grabbed mine, and we walked at her pace up the driveway toward Marg's house. Once inside, I found her Barbie bathing suit in our bag and put it on her. I pulled her towel out of the bag, wrapped it around her shoulders and sent her out into the back yard with instructions to wait for me. Then I went into the main floor bathroom and changed into my swim shorts.

When I went into the back yard Dana was sitting under the awning with Marg and Laurie, beside the natural gas fire pit. Norm was shirtless, burning his back, and doing his medical charts at the picnic table on the upper tier of their huge cedar deck. It was a great day to be in their back yard, which served as a focal point for family gatherings all summer long. It was probably Dana's favourite place to be, especially in the large swimming pool. There was so much to do in this yard and Dana's activity level always intensified here.

It was a warm comfortable day with little wind or cloud. Dana and I finally got into the water, which Marg kept at about 90 degrees Fahrenheit. The family picked on Marg about this habit, but she shrugged us off, noting that the kids liked the pool warm.

Dana's skills in the water had improved tremendously. By now she could take a breath and swim to the bottom of the deep end of the pool, which was about eight feet deep. She and I would put on goggles and play Atlantis. This was a game where I was a sea monster from Atlantis, usually with a pirate's voice and Dana was, of course, a mermaid, preferably Disney's Ariel. Normally, Dana could swim for hours. She was a natural swimmer and moved through the water with agility and control.

We had been in the pool for about half an hour when her

energy began to wane.

"Tired, Daddy," she gasped, breaking the surface in the shallow end after another long trip back up from Atlantis.

"You're tired? We've only been in the water a little while."

"Oh, Jim, we didn't feed the kids any lunch yet," Laurie reasoned.

"What time is it?" I asked.

"It's about 1:30 pm," Marg responded.

Laurie got up and made her way to the back door, which was close to the kitchen. "Do you want anything?" she asked, looking at me.

"No. Just a beer I guess," I answered.

Laurie and Marg prepared some sandwiches and drinks, and brought them out poolside. While they were at work, I got out of the pool and held up a towel beside the ladder for Dana as she climbed out of the pool. She wrapped herself in it and sat down in a lawn chair beside the fire to warm up. Laurie brought Dana a plate with a ham and cheese sandwich, Coke, and some cookies. I noticed that the tray of lunch goodies was missing something, so I went back inside to the fridge and grabbed Norm a beer as well.

Laurie and I sat down in our chairs, which were about 20 feet away from Dana. Dana stared trance-like at the fire, as she slowly lifted the sandwich up to her mouth and let it down from time to time.

"Something's wrong with her. What is it?" Laurie asked as she reached for my hand.

"I don't know. She's probably fine," I responded in an attempt to calm her worries.

"Have you brought her in to see someone yet?" Marg inquired.

"Yes, I brought her to see Al a few weeks ago. He looked for a urinary tract infection, but the results came up negative."

Norm looked up from his charts, after quietly listening to the conversation for a few minutes. He looked at Dana and then looked back at us.

"She's fine," he said. "She's growing. Quit worrying about nothing. She's fine." With that, he put his mind back on his charts and continued on.

"Don't listen to that quack," Marg barked, loud enough for Norm to hear.

Laurie leaned her petite body into my shoulders and looked at the cedar deck.

"What should I do, Mom?" she asked.

"Just keep watching her closely. If there's something wrong, you'll know."

I put my arm around Laurie's shoulder and watched Dana, while listening to the remainder of the conversation. Dana didn't say anything. She just slowly ate her food and drank her Coke. When she was finished, she sat beside the fire with the blanket wrapped around her and watched the blue natural gas flame dance skyward through the old lava rocks arranged on the fire pit grill.

The conversation between the four adults carried on. After some time, Dana stood up, went inside, and turned on the TV. I listened to the talk for a few more minutes and then went in to see how she was. She was attempting to put in *The Lion King* video.

"Do you need some help?" I asked her.

She thought for a few seconds and then answered. "No, I can do it."

I watched her, and sure enough, after some experimenting, she was able to orient the video properly, push it into the VCR slot, and press play. She turned the TV to channel three and turned up the volume.

"See, Daddy? I can do it," She beamed proudly.

I rubbed her blonde hair and stood up to go back to the conversation outside.

"You're a smart girl. Good job."

After about 20 minutes, I peeked inside the sliding living room door and saw Dana curled up under a blanket sleeping. I went back to my chair.

"Is she alright?" Laurie asked.

"She's sleeping," I answered.

"She doesn't take naps in the afternoon anymore, does she?" Marg asked.

"No. But she's starting to again," Laurie responded. "I don't know. I know that I'm a worry-wart, but she's not herself right now."

"Yes, you are a worry-wart," Norm stated, looking up from his charts again. "She's been swimming hard on no lunch. She's just tired."

"Be quiet, Dad!" Marg ordered.

The afternoon faded, and soon it was 4:00 pm. Laurie and I packed up the wet swimming things, put them into a grocery bag from Marg's closet, and I loaded it into the minivan. I woke up Ross, brought him downstairs, and loaded him into his car seat in the van. He protested loudly. Laurie woke Dana and strapped her in her booster seat. She protested loudly. Marg and Norm laughed and waved goodbye as we drove off to my parents' house in our minivan amid the screams of kids roused too soon.

We drove across St. Albert and in a few minutes arrived at my parents' house. We unloaded the kids, brought them into the house, and cut them loose. I went back to the minivan and grabbed the wine. My parents, Ray and Judy, were already serving hors d'oeurvres of spring rolls, fresh salsa and nachos, and spicy Murphy's meat with cheese and crackers. We all kidded Judy about the size of the meals that she prepared. No one needed that much food. By the end of her meals there were lots of leftovers and everyone had eaten too much. I had three siblings, an older sister, her twin brother, and a younger sister. All were married. My older sister had three children.

My family was close, smart, and stubborn, but quiet in many ways. Ray and Judy were generous, caring, and did their best to give whatever they had, even when times were tough for them. Judy and my sisters were actively involved in the Lutheran Faith and Ray, my brother, and I were not.

Dana and Ross had joined in on playing with the other kids as soon as they'd calmed down sufficiently from the minivan ride. The kids went into the back yard to play a dress-up game with the sheets and assorted clothes they'd pulled out of Judy's play box. I sat at the kitchen table, and joined in the conversations with the other adults. Both Laurie and I diverted our attention to the backyard as Dana's crying intensified. "Give me back that dress Dana!" Annika, my older sister

Susan's daughter demanded.

"No! I had it first. Go get another dress."

"You didn't have it first. I did!" Annika returned as she tightened her grip on the dress and pulled much smaller Dana over face-first onto the grass.

Laurie got up and went outside with Susan close behind.

"What's going on here?" she asked.

Dana got up from the grass and ran to Laurie.

"Annika won't give me the dress that I had," she replied.

"But I had it first Aunty Laurie," Annika protested.

Susan turned to her eldest daughter, Caitlin. "Who had this dress first Caity?"

"I didn't see, Mom."

Laurie grabbed the dress from Annika. "If you two can't solve this yourselves, then nobody will get this dress."

Laurie took the dress inside and laid it over one of the chairs. Annika moved on to another activity, but Dana chased Laurie into the house, now screaming.

"No! No, Mommy! I had that dress first! Please give it to me!"

Laurie turned and stopped Dana from taking the dress again. "I've made my decision, Dana. You can't have that dress. Go do something else."

Dana screamed louder, grabbed a nearby cushion, and threw it against the wall. "That's one, Dana. If I get to three and you haven't started to behave properly, I'm putting you upstairs for a timeout."

Dana had now become more irrational, and was crying and screaming inconsolably. She looked around the room, presumably for something else to throw, and decided to make another run for the dress. Laurie stopped her by grabbing her arm.

"That's two, Dana. You're making Mommy angry."

Dana screamed again and punched Laurie in the leg. "That's three. That's it, you're going for a timeout."

Laurie picked Dana up, who was now kicking and screaming in a fit. She carried her up to the spare room at the top of the stairs and put her on the bed.

"Don't come out of there until I come and get you!" Laurie ordered while closing the bedroom door forcefully.

"No! I won't stay in here. No!" Dana yelled, jumped off the bed, and violently swung the door open.

Then she folded her arms and stood in the open doorway.

"If you don't get back into that bed, Mommy is going to spank your bum," Laurie sternly warned Dana.

"No! I won't get into the bed," Dana screamed.

Laurie bent down, spun Dana around and slapped her bottom. Then she picked her child up and put her back into the bed, demanded that she stay for her time out, and closed the door again. Dana screamed, got out of the bed, and again flung the door open."

"Jim," Laurie yelled down the stairs. "Please come help!"

"What the hell is going on up there?" Judy inquired, sitting at the kitchen table with me.

"I don't know," I huffed as I put my drink on the table, pushed back my chair, and stood up to walk up the stairs. "But here comes Daddy the hammer."

At the top of the stairs Laurie met me. "You're not always

the hammer. I actually do most of the disciplining with these kids while you're at work. I've run out of options in this case. Are you going to help me here or just bitch about having to participate in your kid's upbringing?"

"Yes, yes. Just go downstairs," I grunted.

I swung the door open and went to pick Dana up. She was still crying and yelling. I tried to pull her close to comfort her before talking to her about the situation. "How's my Dana Banayna?"

Dana slapped my face. "I want Mommy! Put me down!"

"Listen girl. You've had your chance with Mommy. Now you have to talk to me," I scolded her as I picked her up, threw her back onto the bed, left the room, and closed the door.

"Don't be so rough with her," Judy instructed me from the bottom of the stairs.

The temper tantrum grew in intensity and volume. Dana did not open the door this time, but her screams became chest deflating and she was making herself hoarse. There were sounds of moving furniture coming from the room. I listened and thought about it for a few moments, trying to cool down. Then some loud thumps could be heard through the door.

"Get in there, Jim!" Laurie begged, listening to the actions play out from the bottom of the stairs, with Judy standing beside her.

"This isn't a spectator sport you two!" I barked as I opened the door again.

"Dana!"

Dana was still screaming. She looked up at me and threw the spare diapers across the room toward the door. Dana, all 35 pounds of her, had pulled the mattress off the single bed and onto the floor. She had flipped the portable playpen, pulled the drawers out of the chest of drawers, and was working on pulling the chest of drawers over. I walked in and grabbed her. She was kicking and screaming, and we sat on the bed. I held her tight and close to my chest as she continued to struggle.

"Please stop. Just stop, Dana. It's okay, just stop." I begged, lowering and slowing my voice.

"Shh, shh, shh," I whispered soothingly into her ear.

Dana's screams slowly turned into sobs. She finally stopped struggling and buried her head into my neck. As she began to speak her sobs left her voice vibrating.

"Daddy, I just wanted that dress. Could you please get it for me?"

I thought for a long moment about that question, not wanting to restart her tantrum, but also not wanting to give in to her tantrum. "Why don't we go down and look through Grammy's things for something just as good as that dress?"

Dana pulled back from my neck for a few seconds and wiped her eyes with her forearm. "Okay, Daddy."

Then she leaned back in and hugged me. When the embrace was complete, I lifted her gently to the ground, extended out my right hand and led her down the stairs, past Judy and Laurie and all of the other silent onlookers to explore the toy box in the laundry room. All that it took was the first dress that I found and picked up.

Dinner was served shortly thereafter. No one talked about the incident at first. There really wasn't anything to say.

CHAPTER 4

Friday July 7, 2000

I had been waiting for this day for what seemed like forever. We were going someplace new for the annual McDonald family camping trip. Bill had found a new campground for us at Lesser Slave Lake during his travels in Northern Alberta. Martin River Campground on the northeast shore of the lake sounded perfect for our group.

Bill, Kim and their kids made the three hour drive to the campground on Thursday night so that Bill could reserve enough good interconnected camp sites for our entire family.

I left work a little after noon. The morning hadn't gone by fast enough. Work was starting to increase in intensity, bringing added responsibility, pay, and prestige, but also stress. The relationship that my employer, Waiward Steel Fabricators, had with our shop employees' union had deteriorated to an unworkable condition. My good friends, and employers, Ted Degner and Don Oborowsky were struggling to find common ground with the business agent of the union. I had petitioned to step into this situation, knowing how horrible it was, and knowing that it could lead to better opportunities at work for me. My petition was successful. Now, I was reaping what I had sown and Ted and Don were much happier owners.

The drive home from work took only minutes at the quick Friday afternoon lunch pace. I had the local rock radio station blasting the tunes in my ten year old pickup truck, at ease in the knowledge that Laurie had spent the entire morning and night before loading the minivan for the trip. All that I had to do was stop at the liquor store to buy the alcohol and some ice for the coolers.

I arrived at our oddity of an old Sherwood Park bungalow and commenced with the ritual of vehicle juggling. The bungalow had no real front door. The narrow front of the house was filled with large picture windows. This allowed passers by to see almost everything happening on the main floor. The thing that Laurie hated most about the house was that both main entrances were on the sides.

The house was built on a narrow lot, with a two-vehicle garage tucked in behind it and a tremendously long single lane driveway leading past the house to the garage. The garage had two small doors. The garage was built so close to the house that the left door was rendered useless for vehicles, as even small cars could not negotiate the tight turn from the corner of the house. We had bought the house right before getting married and took possession the day after our January 14 wedding. I was 24 years-old and in such a rush to buy that I bought this house even with the various protests of my father. I thought it was perfect, then. After five years of maturing, dealing with the oddities of this house, and seeing better homes that we could afford, I had soured on the usefulness of the house. Dana, however, loved the house. Ross liked the house well enough, but not as much as food.

The minivan was in the driveway and had to be moved to the street. Then my pickup could be parked back in the driveway. Then the minivan could be brought back in behind the pickup. This was an all too frequent pain in the ass. Winter was worse. Shoveling the driveway was horrible with the neighbour's fence tight to the driveway on one side and the long side of the house on the other. There was nowhere easy to shovel the snow. This house would have to go, and hopefully soon.

Ross, Dana, and Sasha were already loaded into the minivan. Laurie had taken out the heavy back seat herself to make room for the dog and all of our camping gear. I loaded the drink cooler into the back of the minivan and packed the bags of ice into the food and drink coolers. I slipped inside the house, grabbed a shower and changed while Laurie and the kids waited in the minivan, singing songs.

The drive to the campground was excruciating for my patience. Dana needed three pee-breaks at various times during the trip up. Ross slept most of the way. Dana was excited to see the deer, coyotes, cows, sheep, horses, and the odd red tailed hawk perched on a telephone pole. Sasha didn't care about any of the numerous animals that we saw as the minivan slipped through the greening Alberta farm country during the afternoon. However, Sasha would explode into deep throaty barks, lunging at the van windows, anytime a dog could be seen. This would continue until I yelled at her to shut up.

We arrived at the campground at about 4:00 pm. The kids sprang out of the van and ran over to give Norm and Marg a hug and hello. Laurie and I went for a quick walk around the site. The campsite that Bill and Kim chose exceeded my expectations. There was a long row of mature poplar and spruce trees separating it from the windswept beach, which would protect our frequent gatherings. The beach was reachable by walking a short path and descending a two-storey, wooden staircase. The beach was several hundred metres of white sand, tough weeds, and ages of storm-brought driftwood in every direction, perfect for an endless array of childhood adventures. The 100-kilometre fetch of the lake came directly at the beach from the west. The result was lots of wind and plenty of waves to play in.

The campsite was comprised of four individual sites accessible by the A and B road loop in the campground. There was a public water tap and outhouse adjacent to the site and a great central metal raised box fire-pit with a hinged grill. This was a provincial campground so the firewood was free, unlike the federal campgrounds in Jasper and Banff, where you pay for everything. Best of all, the individual sites were huge, which would help to disperse the volume of our debates in the middle of the night. There were so many trees and so much space separating the other sites from our four that the illusion of privacy was complete.

Laurie and I took the better part of an hour to set up our tent, blow-up mattresses, and sleeping bags. Our regular suppertime had come and gone. "Mommy?" Dana tugged on

Laurie's shirt, with Ross close behind.

"Yes, Dana."

"Can I have a pop and some chips?"

"Go ahead, honey. The pop is in the cooler. The chips are open on the picnic table."

Dana and Ross turned to walk away and collect their treats. "Hey you two," I demanded. "What do you say to Mom?"

"Thank you," Dana responded, looking down at her feet instead of at Laurie.

Ross simply turned and smiled at us.

"Don't eat too much. Supper's coming," Marg interrupted.

"Okay, Grandma," Dana answered.

Dana and Ross took their treats and went back to playing with Bill and Kim's kids. Marg walked toward Laurie and me. "That's the second pop she's had in about twenty minutes. Don't you think that's too much?" Marg asked.

Norm looked up from chopping wood with his new splitter, "She's just thirsty. Quit worrying. Thirsty! That's it."

"Be quiet, Dad! I'm talking," Marg barked.

"She's not well, Mom. You know that. We still don't know what's happening with her. All of the tests come up negative," Laurie complained.

"Is it getting worse?" Marg asked.

"She seems to be getting worse, but I still don't know what it is," Laurie answered.

"It's hard to tell because we're watching everything she does and maybe we aren't a good judge of what is happening anymore," I added.

"I hope she gets better, whatever it is. Come on, let's go eat supper," Marg said.

We gathered around the fire to cook hot dogs and sausages on long metal forks in the open flames. It was a supreme junk food camp meal. Bill threw me a beer as I came close to the fire.

"You look as dry as the Sahara Desert," he laughed as I caught the beer, opened it, and took a large gulp.

"Thanks, old man," I responded wiping my mouth with my forearm.

The other family members arrived throughout the evening. More drinks and socializing continued by the fire. At about 8:30 pm the adults gathered the kids by the fire and sang campfire songs with them. Marshmallows were cooked on the open flame. I was never much for this type of thing so I politely sat with everybody, without singing. By 9:00 pm the kids were in their sleeping bags. The adults stayed up talking and telling stories about our adventures of late. At about midnight, adults started making their way to their own tents and tent-trailers. The guys, as usual, stayed up the latest, becoming suitably drunk. By 2:00 am, Al, Scotty, Bill, and I were the only ones still up. We'd had our fill of stories, beer, and snack food. It was time for bed.

As I crawled into the tent, Laurie was fast asleep, as was Ross. Dana sat up and looked at me. "I'm thirsty, Daddy."

"Do you want some juice?"

"No. Water."

I hesitated for a moment, lost in the decision of ignoring her and going to bed or dragging my inebriated body out of the tent and back to the water bottle stored on the picnic table.

She asked again and I forced myself to go. All of the lights and the fire were out so I strapped the Petzel light to my head, turned it on, and stumbled through the dark to the picnic table. I returned with a large plastic beer glass full of water. Dana drank it all in a few moments.

"More, Daddy. Please. I'm still thirsty."

I was shocked, but made my way out again and poured her another glass. Again she drank it. My tiny girl of no more than 35 pounds had just gulped a wine bottle worth of water. She hated water! She always had.

"Are you still thirsty, Dana?" I asked.

"No, Daddy," she sighed.

I shone the light into her face when I had asked the question. She was pale and looked tired with dark lines under her eyes. I tucked her back into her sleeping bag and crawled into bed with Laurie. It was about 2:30 am.

The mattress shook as Laurie rolled around trying to get up.

"Mommy. Mommy!" Dana cried.

"What is it, honey?" I asked.

"I have to go pee. I have to go pee badly!"

I looked at my watch. 2:55 am. Laurie rubbed her eyes and looked over at me. "Will you please take her to the bathroom, Jim?"

"Come on, Dana. Let's go," I whispered, leaning over to pick her up, trying not to wake an already stirring Ross. My eyes felt like they were full of beach sand and I struggled to keep them open.

Dana sat down on the kids' porta-potty that was set up by

the outhouse. I listened intently as she urinated for close to 30 seconds without stopping. When she stood up, I was astonished to see the large removable bowl in the potty almost full of urine. Dana held my hand as I lead her back to the tent and into her bed.

This action was duplicated at about 5:30 am. When Dana was done, she drank another beer glass full of water.

Morning came, and I could hear the group gathering around the picnic table and the campfire to prepare their breakfasts. I could also feel my exhaustion and hangover growing. Laurie, Ross, and Dana were sound asleep. I looked at my watch. It was 7:45 am. The sun wasn't yet fully on our tent, which would raise the temperature to uncomfortable heights, so I rejoined my family in sleep. By 9:00 am, I awoke again, and could now hear Bill making smart-assed remarks about me. It was time for me to get up and conduct the beer and back bacon ritual, or at least defend myself. Laurie and the kids remained in bed.

I crawled out of the tent, stretched, and roared. Bill threw me a beer.

"That's disgusting, Bill and Jim!" Marg scolded.

"Jimmy needs it to cook the back bacon," Bill reassured Marg, not fooling anyone as we both opened our beers and gulped.

I opened up my dry storage container, rummaged around and found an old frying pan with little to no T-fal coating left and a large scuba diving knife. Bill, the family's chief procurer of fine meats, produced a two-pound package of AAA Canadian back bacon, complete with corn meal.

The ritual was simple, as it was designed by one of my buddies in high school as a morning excuse to drink beer while camping. One slice of bacon, of ample thickness, could be in the pan at any one time, but only one. Share your beer and share the cooked slices with all who would have some. Cook the bacon in the beer over an open flame. Drink the beer as the bacon cooks. It was a perfect activity and produced a fine morning beer buzz as well as great tasting golden brown back bacon to eat.

The fun continued for some time, much to the disgust of Marg, and possibly others. Laurie and the kids woke up close to 10:00 am. Ross and Laurie tried some of the bacon. Dana yawned and looked very tired. She nibbled at a piece, but tried to pick at a muffin soon after. "Who wants to come to the beach with me?" Christine announced.

All of the kids quickly dressed into swimsuits and beach clothes and gathered around her like she was the Pied Piper. As Christine marched the crowd down the path and stairs toward the beach, the other adults who would be joining her gathered up chairs and beach toys. I had noticed some still water a few hundred feet south from the stairs on the beach. Laurie, Scotty, and Marg had started the breakfast dishes so I left the bacon pan and walked down to the beach after guzzling the remainder of my beer.

Once I reached the bottom of the stairs I called over to the mob playing with Christine.

"Who wants to go on a tadpole hunt with Uncle Jim?"

"Yes! Me! I do! I do!" Dana and Christine's daughter Lauren answered.

"Well come on. Let's go!" I called to them.

They ran over to me and the hunt was on. Our troop walked south on the beach, scouring it for treasures such as wave worn rocks that looked like old Indian arrowheads, drift wood walking sticks, ladybugs, bald eagles sitting in trees, ducks in the waves, and finally tadpoles.

"Look you guys. Tadpoles!" I yelled upon reaching the still water that gathered on the low points of the beach from the little streams feeding into the lake.

The tadpoles were teaming in the tannin-stained, weed-choked water, as were water striders and whirligigs. It was kid heaven, and took me back to when I was a child exploring the still ponds of Northern Ontario. The kids and I talked about the various bugs and animals inhabiting the water, each of us feeding off the others' excitement at seeing new and wonderful things. Soon Scotty joined in the adventure with more kids.

"Daddy?" Dana looked up at me.

"Yes, honey?"

"I'm tired."

"You're tired?" I asked, not wanting to interrupt the fun we were all having.

"I want to go back to see Mommy," Dana demanded.

"Well," I said, looking around once more at the scene. "Can you walk back by yourself?"

"No. You take me."

"Go ahead Jim, I'll stay with Lauren," Scotty offered.

I finally gave in and extended my hand down to Dana. We walked back to the campsite, where Laurie was preparing sandwiches for a hike that we would be going on that afternoon. Ross had already returned from the beach and was with her.

"Can I have some water?" Dana asked.

"Yes, Dana," Laurie answered, pouring her a large glass.

Dana drank it quickly and sat down by the fire. Al was making sandwiches with Laurie at the picnic table. Norm was watching the incident with a look of concern.

"Al, what is wrong with that kid?" Laurie asked, as Norm diverted his attention away once he saw that Al was answering Laurie's question. "Look how skinny and pale she's getting. Can we bring her back in to you next week?"

"Sure," Al responded. "We'll set it up when I get back to the clinic."

"What's wrong with her? Do you think we should test her for a urinary tract infection again?" Laurie questioned.

"We can do that. But, I don't know if that's it. I've been watching her this weekend. It's kind of weird. Maybe she has diabetes."

"Don't say that!" Laurie snapped.

"I'm just joking Laurie. I'm sure Dana's fine," Al reassured her.

Norm looked up from his Dick Francis novel as he sat in a chair by the fire, "She's fine. Quit worrying you idiots."

"Shut up, Dad!" A unified chorus sounded.

Norm looked back down at his novel with a wry grin plastered across his face, satisfied with the diversionary rise he had gotten out of everyone.

CHAPTER 5:

Day 2:
Thursday November 14, 2002

My 20-year-old, annoyingly dependable alarm clock successfully jarred me out of a restless sleep at 7:15 am. Laurie hadn't woken me last night to help. I usually slept soundly, but I was on edge with worry about Dana and a persistent nagging question in the back of my mind. "How could Dana have the flu when we'd all had the flu shot?"

When Laurie got up to go check Dana during the night, my eyes opened and I silently listened to her coaxing Dana to eat and fighting the dipping blood sugar, trying to get it to move toward an acceptable level. The sounds of vomiting and crying throughout the night were heartbreaking.

After beating the alarm clock through several snooze periods, I finally turned it off and staggered to the bathroom to shower. Laurie dressed and went downstairs to prepare breakfast for Ross and Eric, and to greet her nieces Julia and

Lauren at the door. Laurie had been Julia and Lauren's day-home caregiver since their births. Dana wouldn't be going to school again today.

I dressed in my usual work uniform of Levis and a collarless shirt and made my way downstairs to the kitchen. The other kids were gathered at the table eating and carrying on, readying themselves for the bus ride to school or to stay and play at our home. I looked into the TV room and Dana was curled up on the couch under her well worn Teddy Bear blanket, which she'd relied on for comfort since she was born.

"Do you think she's getting better?" I asked Laurie, as I rooted through the walk-in pantry gathering food that I'd eat during the workday.

"I don't know," Laurie answered as she peeled a banana for Eric. "No. I'm too tired to even think about it right now. I sure hope so, though."

I packed my food into a plastic grocery bag and readied to go.

"Bye, you guys. I'll see you tonight," I said to the rambunctious table of kids and turned to give Laurie a kiss and hug. Then I walked into the TV room and picked Dana up. She complained a little, but allowed me to pull her in close for one of her Dana hugs.

"Bye, honey. I hope that you feel better tonight. Try to eat something for Mommy."

"I hope I feel better too. Bye, Daddy," Dana whispered into my ear.

I laid her back down onto the couch and covered her up with her blanket and she again slipped easily into the trance of watching her Sponge Bob Square Pants DVD.

I arrived at work shortly before 8:00 am and the problems had arrived before me. The small problem of the day was that the Chief Shop Steward on the night shift had been conducting union business on company time. The General Foreman on nights had submitted a report to me asking for help in dealing with this matter. More distressing, but more difficult to solve, productivity was down and the entire year had been plagued with a series of structural steel fabrication quality problems that would require solutions costing six figures. The mistakes were understandable, because in this difficult market, Waiward was taking on projects that had elements foreign to our normal areas of expertise. Topping this situation was a stark reality edging closer. Our scheduled fabrication work would run out in only three months. Waiward's normal fabrication market in the oil sands area appeared to be tightening up as the unrest in the Middle East intensified. We were losing money on the jobs running through the shop production department, my department, and there were no significant jobs on the horizon.

I completed a few menial tasks and then decided to escape home for lunch. Just before I turned at the gas station by my house, I remembered that Father Wes would be going for his walk by the Alliance Church, which was only another block east. Some words of encouragement from him would have been appreciated at that point. I could see him stretching as I neared the turn to the church and he waved at me. I turned into the parking lot of the church, rolled down my window, and pulled alongside him before he started out. "Do you need some company?" I asked.

"Why not," He answered in his thick Polish accent.

"Perfect! Let me park and I'll be right out."

"You're not really dressed for a hard walk," He stated, as I got out of my truck and he looked down at my black steel toe capped boots, blue jeans, and Waiward leather coat compared with his track suit, running shoes, mitts, and toque.

I opened up the back of my truck and pulled out a pair of gloves and a wind-breaking winter hat.

"Now I'm ready."

"Good. Let's go," Father Wes returned, beginning to walk north through the parking lot and up Clover Bar Road.

"How's Dana doing?"

"Why do you ask that?" I asked.

"Isn't she always a concern? She's a special needs child. Besides, the two boys are as healthy as horses."

"Fair enough. She's sick right now. I suppose she has a bad case of the flu."

"And how are you doing?" Wes asked.

"I'm fine. Why?"

He looked over at me and smiled. "It's eleven thirty on a Thursday morning and you're walking with me instead of looking after your production department. How are you doing?"

"Do you think God is angry with me?"

Father Wes never broke stride, but pondered the question for a few seconds, watching the white air escape from his nose and mouth into the sub-zero air and gather as crystals on his eyelashes.

"That is too big a question for me to answer. What makes

you ask such a question?"

"It feels like nothing is going right. All the little things are going wrong. Things at work are going wrong and things at home are going wrong."

"You and Laurie are doing alright?" Wes questioned.

"Yes. I guess things could always be better, but we're doing fine. I love her and I believe she loves me. Well, she loves me most of the time, anyway."

"You still have your job?"

"Yes."

"Your kids are fine?"

"Yes. Dana's got the flu right now, but other than that they're fine."

"It sounds like not much is going wrong in your life," Wes said, almost in a lecturing tone. "What are you really worried about, Jim?"

I stopped and looked down for a few moments. Father Wes stopped in front of me and bounced on his toes to keep moving.

"I haven't stepped foot in a church for years. I almost abhor the thought of most organized religion. I haven't read the bible since I was confirmed in the Lutheran church as a 13-year-old. In fact, I can't believe in a how-to manual that was written thousands of years ago. Would that make God angry with me?"

Wes stopped bouncing and thought. "There is no answer that I can give you to that question or to your frustration. Maybe the more important question to ask is, are you still angry with God?"

"What?"

"You heard me. Are you still angry with God?"

"I don't know. Sometimes, I guess I still feel angry. I'm getting older now. My kids are getting older. If I was in trouble, if my family was in trouble again, would God interfere?"

"How can you ask these questions when you fight allowing God into your life? Have you tried to let him into your life since your confirmation?" Wes questioned, raising his voice a little.

"I don't like church."

"It's not about church, or me, or Rome, or the Bible, or anything else on Earth. The issue is what you believe and how you act."

"But I don't know how to act!" I complained.

"This isn't a dance that you learn. It's not a science experiment with only one procedure. You feel guilty about not going to church. But maybe church is only an aid to get you closer to God. Maybe you choose what to get out of church."

I was a little stunned by Wes' strong tone of voice, but I tried to listen intently to the words. "You ask if God would interfere on your behalf in your next time of need. Interfere is a poor choice of word. What you ask is do I believe in miracles? I do. They happen every day. There are things that happen every day that science and logic cannot explain. You must look for them. A better question is do you believe in miracles?"

With that question launched at me Father Wes began his strong walking stride north on Clover Bar Road and I stood still, thinking.

Afterwards, I made my way home for lunch, opened the

garage door, parked the truck and walked in through the back entrance door. When I opened the door, Dana was crying with her head on the toilet seat.

"I'm dizzy, Mommy. It hurts."

"I know, honey," Laurie reassured her and wiped the excess vomit off Dana's face with a warm moist towel.

"Is this what she's been like all morning?" I asked while placing my keys on the dryer and taking off my boots.

Laurie looked up from Dana and answered. "She's still not eating much and is throwing up more. I think her ear infection is getting worse, too. I lowered her morning insulin to fight the lows."

Dana's face was starting to look thin. Dana got up with Laurie's assistance. Her pajamas were starting to sag on her thinning frame and the bags under her eyes were growing. Two full days of vomiting and not eating anything of substance were starting to take a visible toll on her tiny body.

"She looks horrible, Lo. She's still not eating?" I asked.

"I know she looks terrible!" Laurie snapped and then paused. "She's not eating well. She's not drinking well. Nothing is staying in the poor girl. She's even throwing up her antibiotics for the ear infection."

"Have you called someone yet?" I asked.

"I've got a call into the diabetes clinic at the U of A Hospital. I'm just waiting for them to return the call. I'll ask Dr. Couch, or one of the nurses, what we should do."

Laurie and I sat down to lunch after Dana was settled. Then I returned to work for the afternoon. I was worried about the situation at home, but was able to immerse myself in the challenges at work for a few hours, allowing 4:30 pm to come and go. I left work and drove home quickly to be at the dinner table before 5:00 pm.

Dana was still lying on the couch when I arrived home and Laurie, Ross, and Eric had already sat down to eat.

"What did they say?" I asked.

"They said to try to stabilize her blood sugar over the night. If she's not improving, we'll have to bring her in. I described what's been going on and they're worried about the amount of fluid that she's lost already."

"No doubt they are. Just look at her," I added.

We finished supper and I played with Eric and Ross in the TV room. Eric was starting to notice hockey and wanted to play all the time. The Oilers game on TV caught his attention as I flipped channels a little after supper.

"Hockey, hockey, hockey!" he exclaimed.

Laurie stayed with Dana while Eric, Ross, and I went out on the street to play pass with our hockey sticks and a ball. Eric and Ross were put to bed by 8:00 pm and Laurie was still working with Dana.

"Do you mind if I go play ball hockey with the boys tonight?" I asked her.

"No. That's okay. I'll leave Dana's glucometer on your pillow. Please check her when you come home and wake me up."

"Fine."

Ball hockey on Thursday nights was a September to May right for the dads over the past five to six years. Scotty was a teacher at a Sherwood Park high school. Bill, Scotty, a group of Scotty's friends, and I got together each week in the school gym to rough each other up a little in some friendly but competitive shinny, complete with fully dressed goalies. Afterward, we'd go to the bar to tip a few beers, eat some chicken wings, and relive old glories and new pursuits.

I went upstairs to my bedroom, found my soccer shin pads and left for the game. After a full evening of fun, I came home at about 1:15 am and locked all of the doors. I crept upstairs and found Laurie and all the kids asleep. I was hopeful. I stripped and took a shower to remove salt stains from my face. Once toweled off, I dressed in a pair of white boxers, picked up the glucometer sitting on my pillow, and quietly walked into Dana's room. Sasha was awake on Dana's bed and sat up to look at me. Her fur was a mess and she was whimpering a little due to her stomach problems.

I grabbed Dana's finger and poked it for some blood. She didn't wake up. The blood soaked into the test strip and the 20-second countdown commenced. The view outside the window caught my attention while I waited. It was strange, but I enjoyed the quiet moments that I spent in the middle of the night looking in on the kids. It was an overcast and chilly night, but the glow from the streetlights on the undersides of the clouds was pretty. The glucometer beeped. Her blood sugar read 17.8 mmol/l. I walked back into my bedroom and shook Laurie.

"Lo. Laurie. Wake up."

"What?"

"It's seventeen point eight. Do I need to give her something?"

"It's been high since this morning. I can't get it down. She needs fluids because the ketones will be going up and she's getting more dehydrated."

Ketones are the toxic byproduct that your body produces when it consumes its own fat. Ketones must be flushed with liquid. I quietly descended the stairs to the kitchen and looked into the fridge. There was a can of sugar free pop hidden in the back. After grabbing the pop, I turned the lights off in the kitchen and walked back to Dana's room.

"Dana. Wake up. Wake up," I spoke directly into her left ear after lifting her out from under her covers and sitting her sideways, facing me, on my left leg. She rolled her eyes open and then went back to sleep once more.

"Dana," I shook her and spoke into her ear. "Wake Up. You have to drink or we go to the hospital."

"My ear hurts, Daddy," She responded as she pointed at her head slightly behind her left ear.

"You have an ear infection, Dana. Remember? You're taking antibiotics for it."

"I don't want to drink. I'm dizzy."

"You have to drink something, Dana. I brought you some sugar-free pop," I ordered as I put the can into her hands.

Without opening her eyes, Dana took four significant drinks of the pop from the can. I thanked her and tucked her back into her bed. Then I crawled into my own bed. Before drifting off to sleep I said a prayer to myself in silence. I asked God to keep Dana safe and to give Laurie the endurance to deal with Dana's flu. I asked God to keep Eric, Ross, and Laurie safe and healthy. I asked God to heal Sasha. I thanked

God for our home and my job.

"Did she drink?" Laurie mumbled, facing away from me lying on the bed.

"Yes."

"Please set your alarm for an hour from now," Laurie whispered.

I complied and we both went back to sleep.

"Mommy!" Dana cried, waking me after what seemed like two minutes of sleep.

Laurie shot up out of bed as my eyes opened. It was 2:45 am. I sat up in bed to hear what was going on.

"I couldn't make it to the toilet, Mommy."

"Oh, Dana. It's okay, honey," Laurie reassured her and then went to the linen closet to get towels.

"Did she keep anything down?" I asked from the bed.

"No," Laurie answered.

Laurie cleaned Dana again, as Dana cried, much weaker than she was only hours before. She carried Dana back to her bed, tucked her in again, and then returned to our bedroom and turned on the lights.

"What do you think?" she asked, bluntly.

"It's been too long. Can you keep this up?" I responded.

"I'm really tired, but I don't think Dana has anything left. We can't get her blood sugar back to normal and she's getting more dehydrated by the hour. I think we should bring her to the hospital first thing in the morning. What do you think?"

"I agree. Where will you bring her?" I asked.

"I think I'll go to the emergency at the U of A Hospital. If they need to ask the diabetes clinic anything they can walk down the hall."

"Sounds fine."

"I'm going to go try to get some water into Dana so she can flush some ketones and I'm going to sleep with her."

"Do you need me to set the alarm?"

"No. I don't think I'll be sleeping much tonight anyway," Laurie answered, as she left the room and went across the hall to care for Dana.

CHAPTER 6

Wednesday July 12, 2000

"Hey Jimmy, come on. It's non-production time," a Waiward coworker almost sang as he sauntered by my office at 8:29 am.

Waiward's weekly production meeting was held every Wednesday at 8:30 am, and usually ran about an hour. The sun was shining and there wasn't a cloud in the sky. I had just been charged by the Union for unfair collective bargaining. If I could only get through to the union's business agent and get him to budge on our impasse I could even stomach a production meeting and maybe, just maybe enjoy a beautiful day.

"Jim, there's a call from your wife," Tracy, the receptionist, whispered forcefully as she stuck her head through the door of the boardroom and interrupted the meeting.

It had been a rough morning for Laurie and Dana. She'd become increasingly ill since we'd returned from camping. She'd started to vomit that morning and was now in more distress than during the weekend. Her thirst was insatiable.

Laurie had decided to take her to see Al again and I went off to work.

"Okay," I said quietly. "Excuse me guys, I'm going to take this call." I went back to my office and dialed in the line.

"Hi. What's up?"

"Do you think you could pick up a prescription on the way home today?"

"Laurie, I was in the middle of a meeting."

"Jim, your kid is sick, can you get a prescription?"

"Yes. Fine. What prescription?"

"Al looked at Dana this morning and ordered another blood test. He's prescribing medication for a urinary tract infection."

"Is that what it is?"

"I don't know. We'll find out after the blood test comes back, but he's going to start her on it now anyway."

"Where will the prescription be?" I asked.

"At the Save-On-Foods."

"Okay. I'll bring it home tonight. How's Dana?"

"I don't know. Fine, maybe. She's not vomiting now, but she looks horrible."

"This sucks. I'll talk to you tonight, Lo."

"What sucks?"

"Nobody knows what the hell is going on. She just gets worse."

"What do you want me to do about it? I'm doing everything I can!"

"I know, Lo. It's just frustrating."

"Well don't take it out on me."

"Fine. Bye."

I gathered my thoughts again to prepare for another round of bargaining with the union. The main focus at this time was on preparing another offer, and writing it in such a way that I could continue with my practice of distributing a copy to every shop employee thereby showing my every move. It was a time-consuming effort, but it appeared to be grinding the union down. They weren't used to having the employees know everything about the closed-room negotiations. It made it difficult to counter what I was explaining in print. In desperation they had charged me with negotiating directly with the employees. They were hoping to force me to stop informing the employees. The phone rang. It was Laurie again.

"Jim?" Laurie asked sounding flustered.

"Yes it's me. What is it now?" I asked.

"Just listen. Al called me back. He had a hunch when he ordered the blood work on Dana. He got them to test her blood sugar. The results came back positive."

"What do you mean? What's positive mean?" I asked, now alarmed.

"Dana has diabetes," Laurie explained with a cracking voice.

"Do they have to run more tests? Do we need to get a second opinion?" I asked hopefully.

"Al already explained it. He said that I could do that, but that it was no use. The test is accurate. It can only be one thing. Dana is Type 1 diabetic."

I sat silent for a moment and tried to keep from crying. I hadn't cried about anything for years, maybe close to a decade. My little girl was sick.

"What am I supposed to do? Do you need help?" I asked.

"Al has already set it up at the University of Alberta Hospital. You have to leave work and meet me there in two hours."

"What's going to happen there?" I asked, scanning my full day-timer.

"I guess it's like school. They'll help Dana to get back on her feet and will teach us how to care for her. My mom's going to take Rossco. You'd better clear your schedule for the next few days."

"Okay. I'll meet you there," I responded.

"Jim, are you okay?"

"No, I'm Shitty! How are you?"

"I don't know. Worried. I love you."

"I love you too, Laurie. See you in a couple of hours."

I sat at my desk staring out at the parking lot for what seemed like a long time. I got up and went down the hall to Ted Degner's office. He was not only half owner of the company and my boss, but he had been my friend since I was 14 years old playing hockey with his son Terry. If my dad wasn't there, Ted was close enough. "You look like shit, Jimmy. What's up?" Ted boomed through a broad smile as I walked into his office.

"I need a few days off, Ted. Is that a problem?"

"A few days off? What's wrong?"

I sat down at his desk. "I guess Dana's just been diagnosed with Type 1 diabetes. I have to go to the hospital and to what amounts to diabetes school, starting in about two hours."

"Oh no!" Ted grimaced and closed his eyes. "Is she going to

be hospitalized?"

"I'm going to find out there."

"That's absolutely horrible. I'm so sorry for you. Please tell Laurie that our family's thoughts and prayers are with you. Take as much time as you need."

"Thanks, Ted," I said, standing to go.

"Hey Jimmy, you'd better go up and see Donny. You know that his son Shonn is diabetic?"

"Of course."

"Don's also one of the founders of the Alberta Foundation for Diabetes Research. Go let him know."

I nodded and walked up the stairs to Don Oborowsky's office. Don was the other owner of Waiward and had helped me work my way up the corporate ladder at Waiward since I was 17. He also treated me like a son. Dwayne Hunka, my direct supervisor and friend was meeting with Don. "Don? I'm sorry to interrupt. Do you have a moment?"

"What the hell do you want?" Don barked, smiling at me.

"Dana's just been diagnosed with Type 1 diabetes."

Don's normally expressive face went limp.

"That's too bad. You go take care of your family. You and I will talk later. I'm very sorry to hear this."

Dwayne stood up and put his hand on my shoulder. "That's terrible news. Good luck and go to your family."

"Thanks," I said, and then left the office and made my way to the hospital.

Laurie had given me precise directions on where to go. The hospital is a massive world-class medical facility, and is a source of civic pride for Edmonton. Now I was one of the unfortunates who find out why. I walked across the pedway and into the hospital, following Laurie's directions to the basement. When I entered the waiting room of the Pediatric Diabetes Education Centre, Laurie and Dana were already waiting. I walked purposefully across the room, picked up Dana and held her tight. I sat down with Dana still in my arms and reached for Laurie's hand. Laurie and I summoned our strength to absorb what we were about to learn.

One of the nurses showed us into a physician's room. Laurie and I sat down and Dana sat up on the physician's examining bed. Moments later the tall, thin, and soft-spoken pediatric endocrinologist Dr. Couch walked in. He wasted no time in delivering the facts as he examined Dana's data.

"I want to explain something to you both right now so that you clearly understand it. Dana is Type 1 diabetic. There is nothing else it can be so you have to get used to it now and learn to deal with it."

It was put so bluntly and by such a quiet and thoughtful appearing man. It didn't sit right. It didn't feel right. I was expecting to be eased into this. Laurie just held my hand and listened.

Dr. Couch examined Dana while explaining to us what had been happening to her tiny body over the past several months to reduce her to this sickened state. Some unknown catalyst, maybe a virus mimicking the protein makeup of her insulin-producing islet cells in her pancreas, had triggered her body to attack and destroy these same islet cells. Approximately 80 percent of the islet cells were destroyed before Type 1 diabetes was diagnosed. That is why it took so long to diagnose, even though we knew she was sick. He explained how insulin is the trigger for our bodies to properly digest and turn food into useable energy. Without insulin, the body literally starves even with regular eating.

Once Dana's body could no longer obtain nourishment through regular channels, it began to consume her fat energy stores. The byproduct of body fat consumed in this manner is ketones, which are toxic and lethal if the levels rise unchecked. Once the ketones reached problematic levels, Dana's body fought back by trying to flush them, which explained her thirst and numerous trips to the bathroom. She had been through a horrific spiral of deteriorating health that would have culminated in her death had she not been diagnosed.

After fully examining Dana, Dr. Couch gave us a small bit of good news.

"You're fortunate that the diabetes was caught relatively early. Most new diabetics must be hospitalized to stabilize them, but Dana's going to be able to go home tonight as an outpatient."

Dr. Couch went on to explain the training that Laurie and I would go through during the next five days. We would spend a generous amount of time with the registered nursing team who would train Laurie and me how to check Dana's blood sugar levels and how to administer the insulin she needed. We would be trained by a registered dietitian on how to properly feed Dana the right amounts of carbohydrates, proteins, and fats for her to survive and be healthy. Finally, we would meet with the counselor daily to check our progress in dealing with the monumental change to our lifestyle that had just been forced upon us. Dr. Couch would monitor Dana's progress and ours.

That first day brought a mix of emotions and events, both good and bad. Dana was very frightened of the glucometer that was issued to us to check her blood sugar. The lancet hurt her when it augured into her tiny finger to draw the blood necessary to wet the test strip in the glucometer. She was terrified of her first insulin injection, the first of tens of thousands of such injections she would endure over her lifetime.

Her blood sugar was tested at a staggering 43 mmol/l when we arrived at the hospital, which supported the enormous amount of ketones she had in her body, creating the life-threatening ketoacidosis. We learned that her blood sugar should ideally be in the range of five to ten mmol/l and that 15 mmol/l was considered high. The nurse showed us how to dip the ketostix in Dana's urine and to evaluate her ketone levels on the colour chart. Dana had to continue drinking large amounts of fluids to flush the ketones out of her body while the insulin returned her digestive functions to normal.

However, with all of these new and sometimes terrifying procedures to learn and endure came one beautiful effect. Our daughter Dana had been returned to us. Within the hour of the first insulin being injected into her body the positive change became evident. Dana's health was returning.

Laurie, Dana, and I completed the five days of training, establishing a new lifestyle full of procedure and discipline for our family. Timing, discipline, and endurance were huge factors in our life from now on. Dana had to eat and have an insulin shot at 8:00 am every day. She needed a snack at 10:00 am. She needed lunch at noon. She needed a snack at 2:30 pm. She needed supper at 5:00 pm and another insulin shot at the same time. She needed a snack at 8:00 pm. She needed to have her blood sugar checked at 8:00 am, noon, 5:00 pm, and 8:00 pm at a minimum.

Each meal had a prescribed amount of carbohydrates, protein, and fat. The carbohydrates and the insulin amounts were the main balancing factors in this ongoing prescription. Any deviation required vigilant monitoring. Dana required five extra carbohydrates for every 20 minutes of physical exertion. If her blood sugar dropped below 3.5 mmol/l, we needed to give her ten quick acting carbohydrates such as apple juice or Lifesavers to stop her from becoming hypoglycemic, otherwise known as going low. If her blood sugar was below 7.5 mmol/l at 8:00 pm, we had to check it again before midnight to ensure that she had enough blood sugar to last the night without going low. The thought of Dana going low in the middle of the night with everyone sleeping horrified me. She could die if that happened.

If her insulin-carbohydrate combination went out of balance in favour of the carbohydrates, her blood sugar would rise and she would become hyperglycemic, also known as high. When this happened we would have to monitor her ketones, get her to drink fluids, keep her activity level low, and manage her blood sugar until it returned to normal.

We learned about the devastating effects that can result from diabetes that is not or cannot be managed properly. Death, blindness, kidney failure, liver disease, and gangrene, just to name a few, can result over time. It was clear to me that Laurie and I had a deadly serious responsibility to manage Dana's disease properly. If we were vigilant and effective at this, Dana had a good chance to grow up and lead a relatively normal life. If we were lazy and inattentive we would slowly be killing our child. The vast amount of vital information delivered to us in such a short time was overwhelming.

I finally returned to work on Tuesday, July 18 after completing the training. I put in a long day and looked at my watch to find that it was shortly after midnight, and I still had so much work to catch up on. It was difficult to focus on anything. I pushed my chair back from my desk for a moment, looked up at the ceiling tiles, and listened to the sounds of clanging metal and machinery whirring from the night shift in the plant. A question had been festering in my mind, fuelling my anger. I had been in so many conversations during my life where older and wiser people than I had explained to me that God has a reason for everything that happens. What possible reason could there be to give Dana this terrible disease? I needed to voice it out loud to bring formality to the thought, ensuring that God would hear me.

"If you exist and you can hear me, why did you allow this to happen to Dana?" I yelled through the ceiling. "She's an awesome little girl and you've allowed her to get this ugly disease. Why? She did nothing wrong. If our family had to be hit with this, why not me?"

I waited for a response. I'm not sure why, because that is a ridiculous hope, but I did it anyway, almost out of instinct. No response came, of course.

A productive idea did strike me moments later once I'd pulled myself back together. Laurie had been getting me to write a letter to Ross and Dana on their birthday each year. The rules to this process were simple. I could write whatever I wanted for each letter, but they were sealed for the kids to receive in one package on their 21st birthday. It was a lovely gesture and I looked forward to writing these letters. It felt like leaving your child a breadcrumb trail to lead them to the answer of where they came from and who their family was and is. Even though Dana's birthday was not until January 2, it was time to write her fourth birthday letter. She needed to know some of what I was thinking, even if she wouldn't read it for another 17 years.

Date:July 18, 2000
For:January 2, 2001
Dear Dana,

It is 1:51 am and I am at work. This letter is a bit of a departure from what your three previous letters were and what I believe the remainder of your letters will be. I don't know if you can imagine how tired I am, but try to. Try to imagine, or if you have seen me like this, then try to remember what I am like when I am totally physically and mentally exhausted and terribly stressed.

You see, for the last few months this pressure has been building. I have now been in collective bargaining with the union at work since August 1999, almost a year. The Union has just recently charged me with bargaining directly with the employees, which is a fairly serious offense in the eyes of the Labour Relations Board. I am in the midst of preparing my defense. Waiward's yearly quality system audit is scheduled for Thursday and Friday, July 20-21, 2000, and I am not ready for it yet. I have just recently been asked to hire approximately 30 new employees for our shop and there is a labour shortage in Alberta at this time. All of this has been really taxing my physical and mental endurance and I am not sure if I can withstand the pressure for much longer.

Then, something absolutely terrifying happened. On Wednesday July 12, 2000, you were diagnosed with diabetes. My idea of order in my world was completely shattered in an instant and the pressure that I felt before was now infinitely greater. Your mom and I had fashioned a lifestyle that we were now used to and as fast as you can say diabetes, it was gone and we had to begin the adjustment to living a new lifestyle.

Those first few days were very difficult for me. On Thursday July 13, 2000 I had to go into work and call everyone that had deadlines I was supposed to meet and explain to them that I would be late.

The pressure of work was still there even though I thought that I had left it behind to focus on learning how to take care of you. Mom and I were in classes every day, learning new and vital information about the kind of care that you needed. Probably the most difficult thing was putting you through this new and terrifying process of regular blood sugar tests and insulin needles. The look of confusion and terror on your face during those first few days was horrible. Hour after hour, this new reality wore Mom and me down. Mom was always good at letting her emotions go in order to drain and revitalize her, but you know that I am stubborn and tough. I would not give in to this thing and would overcome without breaking down, just like I had overcome every other challenge in my life to that point. Breaking down would be a show of weakness for me.

However, the emotional grind of those first few days was relentless.

Finally, Sunday came. This day was a true test of my abilities as a dad. What you have to understand is that my overall approach as a dad to that point was to remain at an emotional distance from you and Ross. In that way, I could handle all challenges without losing my cool, but I now think that this was probably keeping me from some important learning and experiences with you. During our early learning, the doctors at the U of A Hospital had taught us that you were in danger of hypoglycemia if your blood sugar dropped below 3.5 mmol/l. On Sunday, we were at Grandma's and you swam for hours during the day. We didn't give you anything but your regular meals to counter this extra activity and by supper your blood sugar was at 6.7 mmol/l. I wasn't scared, but was concerned and both your mom and I were very tired by then. We carried on with your insulin shot, but by 7:40 pm your blood sugar was 2.7 mmol/l. I was concerned then. We treated your low blood sugar and shortly thereafter were at home. I stayed up and watched a movie until 11:40 pm. Then I went into your room and tested you again. This time your blood sugar was 2.4 mmol/l and I was very worried. We treated this again and your mom set her alarm for 4:00 am.

I went to bed at about 12:30 am, but did not sleep well and I was exhausted. I was very worried about you going into a seizure while we slept. I can remember dreaming that night about you dying from this. The dream and the corresponding emotions were so real that it woke me at about 2:00 am. Tears were streaming down my face and I couldn't stop crying. I got out of bed and went into the living room where I continued to cry. I know very well that that moment was the first time I truly understood how powerful the bond could be between a dad and his child. That real fear and sense of loss

I experienced on that Sunday night was a huge wake up call for me. It was the first time I knew that I would do anything I could to keep you safe and to make you feel safe and loved. That moment, in the middle of my tears and pain, was the first moment I ever had where I knew with every part of me that I was a father. That was your gift to me in those first few ugly days after learning you had diabetes and I thank you.

You are a wonderful daughter and are a significant part of a wonderful family. I am blessed to know you and to be a part of your life.

I hope that we both grow together over the following year, and I look forward to writing you another letter on January 2, 2002.

Love,

Dad

CHAPTER 7

Wednesday July 26, 2000

"Do you still think it was a good idea not to cancel our vacation?" Laurie asked.

I responded as positively as I could. "Absolutely. What were we going to do at home, mope around and feel sorry for ourselves? Besides, Christine and Scotty had this trip planned six months ago."

"I suppose that Lauren would have been devastated if we didn't come and she couldn't be with Dana," Laurie added.

"She would have been crushed. Besides, the week is going great," I commented.

We were returning to our campsite in the Wapiti campground in Jasper National Park. The afternoon was spent at the top of Whistler Mountain. The gondola ride was fantastic and the kids were blown away by the view and spectacular beauty of the mountains. Ross was a little scared, but he is cautious about safety. Dana had eaten everything that we'd given her. In addition, she had started to allow us to administer the blood sugar tests and insulin needles a little easier than in the days before, with a few exceptions.

The mountaintop was so beautiful that we'd decided to follow Julia's instincts and climb for a while. The kids ran up and down and climbed every large rock before them. It was heartwarming to see Dana's athleticism returning and to see her chasing Lauren everywhere she went. The two moved like little mountain goats. We climbed for about an hour and then Julia picked a spot for all of us to eat lunch. The clear view allowed us to see across the entire Tonquin Valley.

After lunch, we climbed some more and hunted for a look at the marmots moving about the loose shale, exciting the kids by telling them about the king of all the marmots, Whistler, the namesake of the mountain. They searched for Whistler all afternoon, asking each time a marmot was spotted if they'd achieved their goal. The only miscue on the trip was that Laurie and I forgot to feed Dana extra carbohydrates for the activity on the mountain. There was much to get used to in our new lifestyle. Her blood sugar was a little high at lunch, at 18 mmol/l. By the time we'd realized the mistake we were already coming down the gondola. Dana did not appear low and it was only 30 minutes to supper. We decided to watch her and check her just before supper.

"How do you think she's doing with all this?" Laurie asked, as we pulled the minivan into our campsite, beside Scotty and Christine's site.

The question out of the blue took a few seconds to register with me.

"With what?"

"Dr. Couch, the nurses, and the social worker all told us that Dana has been traumatized by all of this and that she doesn't understand what has happened to her. They told us that she will resent us and the staff at the diabetes clinic because the needles and the blood sugar tests hurt. I wonder how she's doing with that?"

I thought about the question for a few seconds. "It's kind of funny isn't it? She was going to die and has now been saved by a medicine that she will hate for the rest of her life. I hope she doesn't hate us. She's probably a little angry though."

"I hope she doesn't hate us. That would be hard," Laurie continued, opening the door to let Ross and Dana out of the minivan.

The four of us made our way over to Christine and Scotty's site to start the supper preparations. Making the fire was a job that I enjoyed immensely and one that I always tried to get when we camped. There's just something therapeutic about splitting wood with an axe and then watching it burn. I cut the different sizes of wood that I'd need to light the fire in the firebox and to keep it burning for a while. Then I arranged the paper and kindling and started the fire. I sat back in the hammock chair to enjoy the warmth and stare into the lapping flames.

"Hey Jimmy, I bought you a day-early birthday present. I understand that with all of us camping in such close proximity you probably won't be getting any this week, so here it is: a new copy of Maxim!" Scotty glowed, as he handed me the cheesy magazine and a cold beer.

"Thanks, old man. Just what I wanted!" I responded,

hoping my sarcasm was dripping.

Scotty just laughed, pulled up a chair beside me, and guided me on a brief tour of the magazine's finer articles and pictures. Laurie and Christine walked behind us, in turn, to peek at the ridiculous pictures and laugh at two grown men getting wrapped up in a rag selling itself as expert on gadgets, sports, beer, chicks, and war.

"Dana, let's check your blood sugar," Laurie called out into the bush where Lauren, Dana, Ross, and Julia were playing.

Dana looked up, but was reluctant to come. "Come on Dana, we have to check it," Laurie called again.

Dana walked slowly over to Laurie and stopped in front of her. Laurie grabbed her hand and pulled it toward her. Dana resisted.

"If you fight this, Dana, it'll hurt more," Laurie explained.

"It hurts my finger," Dana protested.

"I know it hurts, but we have to do this."

Laurie poked Dana's finger with the lancet and Dana cried. She let her go back to the other kids once there was enough blood in the test strip. Christine watched the countdown from behind Laurie, curious to learn more about this new issue in the family. The glucometer returned the reading of 2.9 mmol/l. "We should have given her more food at snack time on the mountain," Christine sighed.

"We just forgot to," I said.

"What do you have to do now?" Scotty questioned.

"We'll give her a juice box for the low and then she can eat supper," Laurie explained.

"She seems a little grumpier than she's been," Christine

commented.

"She was high at lunch and now she's low. The nurse at the diabetes clinic told us that when her blood sugar crashes like that it's hard on Dana," Laurie explained. "Sort of like being punched in the gut."

Laurie treated Dana's low and Scotty, Christine, and I continued to get the steak and corn ready to eat. We prepared the kids' plates first, measuring Dana's plate portions with a scale and her milk with a measuring cup.

"Supper's ready kids," Christine called out.

The kids came running and sat themselves in order around the picnic table.

"Dana, let's do your insulin," Laurie called.

Dana thought for a moment and then folded her arms. We had not tried any other sites for the injections other than the fat behind her upper arms. She fought any attempts to give her the needles in her legs or bum, even though we tried to explain to her that the bum sites would hurt the least. She would only accept her arms as a site.

The clinic staff had spent a good deal of time ensuring that Laurie and I were both competent at cleaning the insulin container, measuring the insulin dose, drawing the dose up into the needle, properly choosing a site, and administering the needle. Dana was skinny, but it was not a good idea to administer the insulin into muscle. If the insulin was injected into muscle it would enter the blood stream too quickly and react too fast. Injecting it into the fat slows the flow of insulin into the bloodstream and results in longer and smoother-acting insulin. One of the only sites on Dana's body with sufficient fat was behind her arms.

In order to get the insulin into the fat behind Dana's arm, you needed to use both hands. You lightly pinched and raised the fat layer up behind her arm in a site free of blemishes or calluses from previous injections and then inserted the needle at about a 45-degree angle. Then, you injected the insulin, pulled the needle out of the site without changing the angle of the needle, and released the pinched layer of skin and fat.

All of this was simple when you tried it on yourself. I had to because I was scared of needles. How could I give Dana needles for years to come if I couldn't do it to myself? So I did it, without fainting.

"No, Mommy. I don't want it," Dana responded, with her arms still folded.

"Dana, you know we have to do this. You have no choice."

"No!" Dana screamed. "It hurts!"

"I know it hurts, honey, but we still have to do it," Laurie coaxed as she gently grabbed Dana's arm, getting the needle ready to inject.

Dana spun violently away from Laurie, accidentally stabbing herself with the needle. She screamed at Laurie and got up from the table. Scotty and I were still in our chairs by the fire watching the scene unfold.

"What do you do now?" Scotty asked me.

"I don't know what we can do. Dr. Couch was pretty clear to us on this issue. We can't let this become a debate. There can be no give. Food, blood sugar checks, and insulin are medicine that simply has to be administered no matter what."

"That's fine, Jim, but what the hell do you want me to do

now?" Laurie shot back. "She's fighting me and refuses to take the shot."

"Fine. I'll do it," I snapped, letting my frustration start to get the better of me.

Laurie handed me the needle and motioned with her arms for me to give it a try. Dana was in our campsite beside our tent whimpering.

"Dana, please let Daddy do your insulin shot."

"No!"

"Dana, I'm very sorry and I know that this is hard, but you have no choice. You need this shot or you will become very sick again."

"I don't care!" Dana yelled at me as I grabbed her arm.

She became hysterical, yelling, kicking and punching me. She called for Mommy. She called for help. She begged me to stop. I sat her on my left knee at the picnic table on our site, wrapped my arm around her to force her to stay on my knee, and held her left arm out. As I pinched enough skin to inject the needle she punched me in the chin with her right hand, slightly jarring me. She continued to violently wriggle her tiny frame until I became afraid of accidentally stabbing her again. I let her go. She scampered into our tent and crawled into her sleeping bag. I stood up and could feel the fury growing in me.

"Let her be for a moment, Jim," Christine urged.

"I won't go through this every damn night! She needs the bloody shot."

I threw the door of the tent open, forcefully unzipped Dana's sleeping bag, flipped Dana over onto her stomach, and I sat on top of her. Dana screamed and begged me to stop. Every muscle in her body was tense and struggling. I pulled her shorts down, pinched the fat on her bum, stuck the needle into the site, and injected the insulin. I left Dana sobbing in the tent, jammed the needle into the biohazard container and sat down to have my dinner.

"That wasn't necessary," Christine said calmly but forcefully.

"Jesus Christ! You give her the damn needle next time," I shot back quickly, grabbed an unopened beer, and walked out of the campsite.

Christine had her arm around Laurie, who was shaken by the incident and Scotty nervously stoked the fire trying not to add any more intensity to the problem.

"I'm going for a walk, Laurie. I'll be back later," I growled, without looking back to see if I was heard.

The sun was already down behind the mountains around Jasper, leaving the cool of the mountain summer evening to set in fully. The fires from the many occupied campsites covered the campground with a silky fog-like blanket and a fragrant burnt wood smell. I could feel tears welling in my eyes and the sandpaper coarseness of my tightening throat as anger gave way to remorse. I fought the urge and kept walking. When I'd walked a few hundred feet farther down the campsite road a clearing opened and I could see a herd of elk. I stopped to watch the magnificent beasts forage, hoping to lose myself in their strength and beauty long enough to cool off.

"Do you want some company to go with that beer?" A voice questioned from my right, near a small fire.

There was a mountain bike leaning up against a tree not far

from the log that the man who had spoken to me was sitting on. The bike had two small panniers on the back. There was no tent set up and there was no food to be seen. His accent was thick, and I knew it from the many Poles that worked with me at Waiward. I was caught off guard by this intervention, but I turned and walked toward him.

"I just might."

"My name is Father Wes."

"What are you doing here?" I asked.

Father Wes smiled and laughed a little. "That's funny you should ask. I don't have to be in church on Wednesday. Why can't I be here enjoying the mountains?"

"I'm sorry. I'm a little distracted right now."

"I imagine that you are. How is your little girl?"

"How do you know about my little girl?"

"Your campsite is only about two hundred feet from this one as the crow flies. She has quite a voice and temper," He replied. "I wonder where she gets it from?"

I looked at my feet for a moment and then sat down next to Father Wes. I opened my beer and offered it to him.

"Thank you very much," Wes said and he took a long full drink. "There is very little better than the first taste of a cold beer."

"I can agree with that."

"So I ask you again. How is your little girl?" Father Wes pressed me.

"She's just been diagnosed with Type 1 diabetes."

"That's too bad. I hope that God will give her the strength to endure this," he said.

"That's just the problem, isn't it?" I jumped in.

"What do you mean?"

"God wouldn't have to give her the strength to endure this if she didn't have the disease."

"I see what you're getting at. Don't you believe that God has a plan and that everything happens for a reason?" Wes argued.

"How did I know that you would say that? Everyone says that. I ask you what good can come from this disease?"

"I don't know what good, if any, can come from this. I do believe that God listens and that there is a reason for all things that happen. You need to have faith. You need to pray for the health of your family and focus on what must be done to keep your family together," he gently argued.

"I don't know where my faith is right now Father. I'm not sure I believe that God does anything to help."

"Be patient, Jim. Have courage. Be strong. Your wife is strong, but she needs your strength too in order to deal with this. Your children need you strong and patient. Enjoy your vacation and thank you for the beer. I will see you again," he concluded, slapping me on the shoulder and handing me the empty beer can.

"Have we met before?"

"Not really. I am at the Alliance Church in Sherwood Park. I know some of your neighbours. Getting to know people is my job. If you would like, you can come and talk to me again. I would like to play a part to help you through this."

"Thank you," I answered, as I got up to walk back to our site. "I'll think about that."

CHAPTER 8

Thursday August 3, 2000

The second week of the vacation was being spent with my uncle Al, aunt Leslie, and their children six-year-old Andrew and three-year-old Emma. Their home was just south of Vancouver in Tsawwassen, British Columbia. It was always a joy for me to spend time with this family because they radiate health and vitality. Time spent with Al and Leslie's family meant time spent on the go with lots to do.

In addition to the time spent being active with them, I had never eaten healthier than when I was with Al and Leslie. Al, now a vegetarian, used to be a real carnivore, but changed his lifestyle after assessing the threat of heart disease in our family. Eating with them meant wonderful vegetarian dishes cooked in inventive ways. However, this was also tough for me, especially being only minutes from the ocean and all of the amazing fresh seafood. As such, today's choice of activity was easy to make. Ross sat at the kitchen table looking out onto the cul de sac. It was 8:15 am.

"Rossco, where do you want to go today?" Al questioned loudly, clapping his two hands together and then rubbing them.

Ross beamed a huge smile and yelled, "Beach!"

"Alright, Rossco!" Leslie encouraged as the rest of the kids danced to the news that we would be going to Boundary Bay.

Dana sat at the table eating corn flakes with banana and milk.

"What was her blood sugar?" I asked Laurie.

"Six point seven," Laurie answered. "Could you please give her the needle so that I can finish my tea?"

"Yes. What do I give her again?"

"Two units of the quick-acting clear H and five units of the long-acting cloudy NPH."

I drew the two units of quick-acting insulin up first and then drew the five units of long-acting. The quick-acting insulin peaked in its effectiveness within the first hour and the long acting peaked within eight hours. This helped to smooth the range of blood sugar values and kept them closer together.

"Come on, Dana. Let's give you your needle," I quietly ordered.

"Not here, Daddy."

"Where?"

"On the couch, away from the table," Dana responded, grabbing her Teddy Bear blanket on the way. She was already developing a ritual to find the courage to deal with the needles. I gave her the shot and she returned to the table to finish her food.

Dana needed 31 carbohydrates in her breakfast to balance with the seven units of insulin. We were discovering that this was a lot of food for a tiny three-year-old. If she was low, she needed ten carbohydrates on top of the 31. In this case, it worked out to a bowl of corn flakes, half a banana, and half of a cup of milk. She finished it without complaint, but was very full.

"She's been eating so much. Does she have to?" Leslie asked.

"I've got a call into the clinic to ask. Maybe we can lower her insulin because this is way more than she used to eat," Laurie answered.

"Why can't you just adjust the dose of insulin based on what she actually eats?" Al asked.

"You can do that, but we're still new so the clinic doesn't want us deviating from this schedule until they're comfortable with our competence in managing the disease," I answered.

"It's frustrating because Dana can't keep this up," Laurie added.

Once breakfast was finished the kids went out to the street to play with the neighbourhood kids. The adults worked in the kitchen to prepare and pack the food, clothes, and supplies that we'd need at the beach. After the two minivans were loaded with kids, gear, and food, Al led us on the short drive through the Tsawwassen streets to one of the playground gems of lower mainland British Columbia, Boundary Bay.

The beach had a few visitors today, but overall it was ours. The kids caught sight of the vast expanse and darted toward it at top speed, with us yelling at them from the rear to stay within eyesight. The bay is shallow and becomes a school of small streams rushing back to sea as the tide ebbs. Thousands of sand dollars, starfish, crabs, tiny fish, and many other forms of sea life can be spotted almost everywhere as the water recedes. The beach called to the explorer in the adults and begged the children to play.

"Dana, it's snack time," Laurie called to the pack of kids chasing some small fish back out to sea.

Dana looked back at Laurie, started to run away again, and then stopped.

"Okay, Mom," she finally agreed.

The other kids followed Dana in and snacks were distributed all around. Dana's morning snack required 15 carbohydrates. Laurie gave her half a cup of fresh locally grown cherries and half a ten-carbohydrate fruit bar. Fruit bars had quickly become a favourite snack for our kids. They were quick, easy, and had ten carbohydrates. Laurie and I didn't treat them like real fruit, which we considered healthier, but we ranked these above cookies and snack food.

Dana and the other kids wolfed down their snacks and ran back into the water.

"Did you put sun screen on the kids?" I asked Laurie.

"We'd better get some on all of us today. It's got to be close to 30 degrees out here," Leslie added.

Al and I grabbed two bottles of the kid's 30 sunblock and chased them down. We gave them all a liberal slathering of the purple gunk. "The wind's picking up nicely," Al called to me in the middle of rubbing lotion on a fighting Ross. "I brought the kite. Should I get it going?"

"Yes! I love your kite, Daddy!" Emma cheered.

"Can you look after the pack for a few moments, Jimbo?"

Al asked.

"No worries."

Al sprinted back to his minivan to retrieve the kite as Leslie pulled her sunglasses slightly down on her nose and gave him a spirited whistle. Inspired, he upped the effort on the return trip, kite in hand. Of course, the kite dancing in the wind, fluttering, and making quick jerky dashes entertained the kids and they begged Al for a turn holding the kite string. He obliged each one and, being a former military helicopter pilot, demanded that each one learn the proper way in which to pilot a properly tuned kite.

"Hey, Al!" Leslie yelled. "Shut down the flight training for lunch. It's eleven forty."

Al reeled in the kite and we herded the pack back to shore for lunch on the blankets and towels. Laurie handed me the glucometer while she doled out food for the other kids.

"Go to the tap over there and wash your hands, Dana," I ordered, pointing at the nearby water fountain.

It was important to wash Dana's hands before doing her blood sugar because sugary residue from past eating could easily sway the blood sugar reading several points, thus giving inaccurate readings that could lead to dangerous decision-making.

"Give me your hand, honey," I asked upon her return and after she'd dried her hands with her beach towel. The reading was 3.7 mmol/l.

"Could I have a juice box, Lo?"

"What's the reading?"

"It's low."

Lunch is the most important meal of the day for Dana and would eventually become the biggest, the one counted on to fill her gas tank with energy so that she could function into the evening. She needed 31 carbohydrates for lunch. Lunch on this day consisted of a ham and cheese sandwich with a little mayonnaise. The two slices of bread counted for 15 carbohydrates each and the mayo added a few more carbohydrates. I took a little sip out of the juice box that I gave her to treat the low. Then she would only drink about 80 ml of the apple juice, which would be ten carbohydrates.

"What do you guys think about going on a walk out to where the sea hits the beach?" Al invited.

"That's got to be about a kilometre out there," Leslie reminded Al.

"It's not that far," he argued.

"I can do it, Daddy," Dana said, grabbing my arm to ensure that I heard her.

"Should I take Rossco?" I asked Laurie.

"I think Rossco and I will play a little closer to this beach."

"I think I'm staying here, too," Leslie stated.

"We want to go, Dad," Emma and Andrew begged.

"That's it then, we're off to where the real ocean meets the beach!" Al enthusiastically ordered his troop.

We were off on a grand adventure. The kids were excited and every creature they came across was a mystery to be solved. Each receding stream was a river to be explored to find its termination. It was pure joy for me to experience. Dana was so happy and her smile was broad. It was infectious and pulled me in to play with them at their elementary level, to explore the bottom of every crab, to wonder aloud the mystery of every empty shell.

We walked and explored for the better part of two hours and were only a few feet from the real ocean. The kids could sense the end of one part of the journey and ran to meet it head-on. The obvious point to terminate the first half of the adventure and start the second half was at the large black and white buoy at the edge of the beach. The pack ran for it.

"Daddy, I feel funny," Dana whined, as she sat in the water and sighed.

"What's wrong, Dana?"

"My legs feel hot," Dana responded.

"It's hot and sunny out today, Dana," I explained.

"No, Daddy. Not that kind of hot. My legs are hot inside. My knees feel funny. I'm tired," she added.

Al ran back to us. "What's wrong?"

"Dana feels funny," I answered, and then provided him the full response. We thought about it for a few seconds.

"Do you think she's low?" Al asked.

"I don't know. She ate a full lunch, but we're running pretty hard out here. Maybe she is. Crap! I forgot to bring any food out with us. She's been running hard for almost two hours. She's supposed to have five carbs for every twenty minutes of hard activity. She could be almost thirty carbs short!"

"You'd better get her back to the beach," Al ordered.

I picked Dana up and hoisted her onto my shoulders.

"We're going to jog a little to get back to the beach. Okay, honey?"

"Okay, Daddy."

I covered the near kilometre in about ten minutes with Dana bouncing on my head. She would have normally loved the ride, but had become lethargic and quiet, which heightened my anxiety and quickened my step.

"What's wrong?" Laurie asked as I ran up the beach and laid Dana onto the towels.

"Dana thinks she's low," I huffed.

Laurie cleaned her hand off with the towel and poked her finger quickly while I sat down on the nearby log and caught my breath. The glucometer reading was 2.2 mmol/l.

"Wow, that's really low!" Leslie remarked.

Laurie treated the low with 15 carbohydrates of apple juice. It was close enough to 2:30 pm to give Dana her afternoon snack of 25 carbohydrates so Laurie doled out 15 carbohydrates of strawberry licorice and ten carbohydrates of fresh cherries for Dana and Ross. Ross could already sense the special treatment that Dana was getting and demanded to be treated the same.

Al, Emma, and Andrew made it back to the beach about thirty minutes later.

"I think we should get home, get the kids settled and make some supper," Leslie suggested, looking a little concerned.

"That sounds good," Laurie agreed.

Ross was playing great and protested wildly as we left the beach to go to our temporary home. The two minivans made quick work of the trip back to the house and the four adults unloaded the gear into the home. The kids went calling on the neighbourhood kids once more as we gave them last minute instructions to stay in the cul-de-sac where we could see them. Leslie made her way into the kitchen and began unloading food from the fridge onto the counter. Al slipped by her and pulled out three beers for Laurie, me, and him. Then Al and Leslie began the simple but elegant process of making two vegetarian pizzas while simultaneously explaining the nutritional value of each topping. The one choice that caught my eye was the Yves vegetarian pepperoni. I asked about it and Leslie gave me a piece. I was instantly hooked. It had all of the spicy pepperoni flavour without any of the heavy fat taste in regular pepperoni.

Al lit the barbecue and in short order the two heaping vegetarian pizzas covered with cheeses, pepperoni, peppers, mushrooms, and tomatoes were on the barbecues with tinfoil underneath. Laurie went outside to call the kids in for supper.

A few moments passed and then the pack stampeded into the house to wash up and jostle for prime table seating.

"Dana, let's do your blood sugar," Laurie ordered.

Dana whined a little and left her chair to go into the living room.

"What's the reading?" I asked.

"Oh man! It's seventeen point four," Laurie answered, obviously frustrated.

"What a huge swing!" Al remarked, as he set the table.

Laurie placed a call to the diabetes clinic. Dr. Couch gave us permission to give Dana an extra half unit of the quick-acting insulin if her blood sugar was above 15 mmol/l. Laurie measured out the 0.5 units of quick acting and 1.5 units of long-acting insulin and debated with Dana for several minutes about the need to take the needle.

"She's so cranky when she's high," Laurie remarked after finishing with the needle. Dana returned to the table a little upset.

The two families ate and traded stories from the day's adventures. Dana needed to eat the full 31 carbohydrates, even though she was high. Laurie took her best guess on what size of a slice of pizza would contain about 15 carbohydrates. Dana drank a half cup of milk, worth six carbohydrates, and then had a little ice cream for dessert, worth ten carbohydrates.

After dinner, the kids asked to watch *Beauty and the Beast*. Al set them up in the living room with blankets, lights out, and the movie running. The adults stayed at the kitchen table catching up with the current events of our lives and cleaned up the dishes, all while having a few drinks.

The movie ended just before 8:00 pm, which was bedtime snack. The kids paraded into the kitchen and sat at the table while Dana washed her hands. Laurie did Dana's blood sugar, which read 4.6 mmol/l.

"That's not enough to get through the night," Al commented.

"No," Laurie responded. "How much extra should we give her?"

"I don't know, Lo. We've been packing food into this kid like she's a cooler for God's sake. How can she continue to eat this much?" I complained.

"Try ten again," Laurie sighed.

"That doesn't sound right," I argued.

"What do you mean it doesn't sound right? How the hell do you know? You decide then!"

"Take a pill! It's got to be more than ten. That's all I'm saying," I added.

"Fine! How much do you think?" Laurie barked.

"More than ten. She's been low by midnight every night since we've been here. Then she screams bloody murder when I wake her up to feed her and she refuses to eat. I want one night this week where she has enough gas to make it through the night," I argued.

"I hear you. How much then?" Laurie pressed.

"Twenty," I offered.

"You feed her," Laurie concluded and turned her head.

"I'll help you," Al stated. "How many carbs does she need for this snack now?"

"Forty," I answered.

Al and I thought for a moment and then came up with the winner. We'd make her a milk shake. Al brought out the blender and set it up. Leslie dug out peach ice cream, measured 15 carbohydrates worth, and scooped it into the blender. I poured half a cup of milk into the blender. Al grabbed a banana and sliced it into the blender to round out the 40 carbohydrates. The shake was ridiculously huge for Dana once mixed. She loved the idea and sat at the table to tackle the enormous of mixture as the other kids ate their smaller snacks.

"I'm full, Daddy," Dana complained about two thirds of the way through the shake.

"You've got to eat it all, honey."

Dana reluctantly agreed and kept eating for a few more minutes until roughly 80 percent of the shake was gone.

"Daddy, I can't eat any more," She begged.

I looked over at Laurie for assistance and she raised her arms indicating that she had no advice to offer.

"Five more bites, Dana," I urged.

"Okay, Daddy."

Once Dana had finished, Laurie dressed the kids in their pajamas and read all four kids a story. Afterward, I brushed Ross and Dana's teeth. Once all four kids had been tucked into bed, the four adults gathered at the kitchen table to play Trivial Pursuit and visit some more.

"That was a ridiculous amount of food for that kid," Laurie stated.

"Yes, but tonight Jimbo and I are going to win," Al added.

"What do you mean?" Leslie asked.

"Every night Jim and I have been up testing that kid at midnight and every night she's low. It's absolutely heartbreaking trying to force food down her throat in the middle of the night. She screams and fights us at every move. Tonight we stuffed so much food in her that she's going to sleep through the night," I explained.

"I hope so," Laurie concluded as we immersed ourselves back into the men versus women trivia competition.

The game concluded, as it should have, with Al and I obnoxiously victorious and the ladies readied for bed. Al and I lingered at the table to drink a beer and talk about life. At about 12:30 am we looked at each other knowingly and decided it was time to test Dana. The house was quiet as the two of us walked silently through the hall to Ross and Dana's bed. I readied the glucometer and inserted the test strip.

"I sure hope we don't have to wake her up again," Al whispered as he watched the procedure.

I gingerly picked up Dana's arm, rolled it over to gain

access to her fingers, and poked the underside of her left thumb. She stirred and Al grimaced. She didn't wake. I slowly applied pressure to the thumb to draw the blood out. Dana rolled her head to the other side. The test strip was placed into the gathering drop of blood and the strip soaked it up. The glucometer beeped indicating enough had gone in. Al and I shuffled out of the room and into the kitchen. We laid the glucometer on the table and counted down the 20 seconds in our head, praying it could not be below 7.5 mmol/l. Al put his hand on my shoulder.

"Come on! Give the kid a break. Don't wake her up tonight," he whispered forcefully.

The glucometer beeped: 12.8 mmol/l.

"There is a God!" Al quietly cheered as he placed his hands together.

"Oh man, that's a relief," I added.

Al went to the fridge and pulled out two more beers. "Boy, you and I need to celebrate!"

We sat at the kitchen table, drank the beers, and traded stories of diabetes and our week fighting Dana's midnight lows together. I placed Dana's log on the table and entered the day's insulin injections and blood sugar readings for Laurie. It was one of the points that really struck me from the clinic. One of the nurses explained that a complaint many diabetic children had about their parents once the child grew was that they had not kept good records of their disease. Laurie had already instilled that discipline into our program so that Dana wouldn't come to that conclusion about us.

The day was now nearly over. I felt useful and good, even

though I knew that morning would come soon. We would have to do it all over again.

CHAPTER 9

Day 3:
Friday November 15, 2002

"Hey Jim are you coming for a drink after work?" A coworker asked at about 2:45 pm as he leaned on my office doorframe.

"Where?" I asked, thinking it would be nice to visit with the other employees.

"I think it'll be at Fargo's," he responded.

"Fair enough. I'll be there."

"How's your day been so far?" he inquired.

"Just wait a second. Can I get this?" I asked, looking at my ringing phone.

He gestured to go ahead and he left to round up more people for the Friday afternoon social.

"Hi, Jim," Laurie said. "Do you think you can come down to the hospital?"

"Sure. What's wrong?"

"I've been here since early this morning and it looks like

we're going to be here for a while longer. It would be nice to have some company," Laurie complained.

"You're still there! Her flu's that bad?" I asked, somewhat shocked.

"It's not the flu. They're checking her for mastoiditis," Laurie explained. "She's already had a CT scan."

"A what scan?" I asked, not sure I heard her correctly and not sure I wanted to.

"A CAT scan," Laurie clarified by using the lay term.

"I'll come right away. Are the kids taken care of?"

"Yes. I called my mom this morning. She's taking care of the kids at our house."

I hung up the phone and went into Ted Degner's office where Ted and his son Terry were having a discussion.

"I've got to take off if that's alright with you guys."

"What's up?" Terry asked.

"I've got to go to the U of A Hospital. I guess Dana doesn't have the flu. They've already done a CAT scan on her looking for mastoiditus."

"What the hell is mastoiditus?" Ted asked.

"I don't have a clue. I'm going to find out."

"That doesn't sound good. Good luck, Jimmy," Ted concluded, sending me off.

I quickly ended my workday and rushed out to my truck. I recklessly negotiated the icy early winter streets to get to the hospital as fast as possible and ran into the emergency, following Laurie's instructions to find her. Dana was asleep when I arrived. My sister Susan and her daughter Annika were sitting with Laurie, keeping her company. I could tell

Annika was disappointed at not being able to talk with Dana. I remained politely quiet and visited with Susan, Annika, and Laurie, waiting to ask Laurie the harder questions to get a fuller update. Finally, not able to wait another minute, I begged Laurie for some answers.

"Tell me about the day. When did you get here? How was she this morning? What's happening?"

"You saw how she was last night. She vomited all night and ate nothing. She couldn't keep any drink down. She was worse this morning. She was totally dehydrated and listless. I only gave her half her normal morning insulin and no quick-acting. When I checked her ketones this morning they'd elevated even more. It confirmed what we talked about last night. I had to bring her in."

"Poor thing," Susan added, stroking Dana's covered leg.

"Is Dana really sick?" Annika asked, pulling on Laurie's leg.

"They don't know for sure yet Annika, but they think she might be," Laurie responded.

"I'm a little sick, too. That's why I'm here," Annika added, smiling.

"When did you get here?" I asked.

"I left home a little after eight. Just as I was leaving the diabetes clinic called. They were happy that I was taking her in once they'd heard the state she was in. I think Dana and I got to the emergency at about eight forty."

"Is your mom going to be fine with the kids if Dana stays over night?" Susan inquired.

"I'll go home later so Marg can go home," I answered.

"Can Dana have a sleepover?" Annika asked Aunty Laurie.

"Not this week Annika," Susan interrupted. "Maybe when she's better."

"So what happened when you got here? Why did she need a CAT scan?" I asked.

"I guess the first doctor examined Dana about thirty minutes after we got to the emergency. He was an intern and examined Dana thoroughly. Then he grilled me about her recent history. Something must have seemed wrong to him. About a half hour later a second doctor came and re-examined her."

"What were they looking at?" I pressed.

"I think Annika and I are going to go. We've heard this and you two could use some time alone," Susan jumped in.

"Bye, Dana," Annika whispered to the still sleeping Dana.

"Good luck sweetie," Susan said as she gently wiped Dana's forehead and then left.

"Bye, Susan," Laurie and I said.

"What were they looking at?" Laurie focused on my question. "Oh, the doctor was concerned about Dana's pain over her left ear. She said it was too intense. I didn't understand her concern because I thought that Dana was just dehydrated from the flu. I seriously thought the pain over her ear was just the ear infection."

"Is this the mastoiditus part?" I asked.

"Yes."

"What the hell is mastoiditus?"

"The mastoid bone is a little soft bone behind your ear. The doctor ordered a CAT scan to see if she had mastoiditus. It's an inflammation of her mastoid bone."

"So is it mastoiditus?" I asked.

"The ENT doesn't think so. He's wondering why everyone is even looking for it. He actually got a little grumpy at the staff for even suggesting it. That's not the worst of it. Dana's blood sugar started to drop fast during the morning. I tested it when they brought her back from the CAT scan and it was three point one. I asked the nurse if I could feed Dana. She said no."

"Why?"

"Because she might need surgery. I told the nurse that she needs to set up an IV or Dana will drop dangerously low. I told him if he didn't do it I would feed her anyway."

"Did he do it?"

"Finally he did at about one," Laurie answered.

"If it's not mastoiditus can we go home?" I asked.

"I already asked the ER doctor and she said that Dana has to stay for now because she still has unexplained pain even though the ENT doesn't think it's mastoiditus."

Dana opened her eyes for a moment and noticed that I was there.

"Hi, Daddy," she mumbled.

"Hello, Dana-Banayna. How do you feel?" I asked.

"Sick," Dana replied, closing her eyes again.

"Oh, then at three Dana was hungry. I asked the nurse if I could feed her because I thought there was no mastoiditus."

"What did the nurse say?"

"He told me no again and that I'd have to wait to speak to the neurosurgeon."

"A neurosurgeon?"

"I have no idea why I have to speak to the neurosurgeon," Laurie added.

"Maybe this is him?" I stated, looking at the new face coming into our room in the ER.

The neurosurgeon introduced himself and quickly briefed Laurie and me about the results of the CAT scan. He explained that there was an indication of air bubbles under Dana's skull, which obviously shouldn't be there. He thought that it might be the work of an anaerobic infection.

Shortly thereafter, a growing team of specialists with long Latin-sounding titles surrounded Laurie, Dana, and me. An infectious disease specialist came on board the growing team. The ENT returned, the neurosurgeon, and a pediatric endocrinologist appeared to care for Dana's diabetic needs. Finally, an anesthesiologist showed up and started asking questions.

"There's an awful lot of horsepower gathering here," I whispered to Laurie.

"I noticed!" Laurie added.

Next the ENT and the neurosurgeon argued their views on the diagnosis and the potential need for surgery. We were not excluded from seeing this. Laurie and I assumed that Dana's problem was moving fast enough that pleasantries might not be important now. The neurosurgeon argued that the team had an urgent need to perform surgery and the ENT argued against this, saying it was premature. Finally, the neurosurgeon came to talk to Laurie and me again.

"What's going on?" Laurie asked nervously.

"She's got a bug," he replied, simplifying for us.

"What do you mean, a bug? What kind of bug?" I asked.

"It's an infection. We don't know what it is yet or where it has gone," he explained.

"What are you going to do next?" Laurie asked.

"She needs to go for an MRI. We're also going to need to do a myringotomy while she's under," he added.

"She's going to be put under? What's a myringotomy?" I asked, as my concern heightened.

"That means they're just going to put tubes in her ears," Laurie reassured me.

The neurosurgeon also tried to calm me.

"Don't worry about Dana being put under general anesthetic. MRI's take too long for a little girl to sit absolutely still. While she's under we'll put the tubes in her ear."

While the neurosurgeon was explaining more of the procedure to us Dana was being prepped for the procedure. It was quite a sight to see the number of tubes coming out of Dana's arms, even if one was feeding her and controlling her diabetes.

"We're also going to take some fluid samples from her left ear while she's under and send that to the lab," the neurosurgeon explained. "Then they'll see what bug she's got."

Forms to sign showed up as the neurosurgeon was completing his explanation. I didn't read anything. I don't think Laurie did either. The only decision to make was yes or no to the procedure. There really was no decision. Laurie signed quickly. It was only an MRI and ear tubes, but Laurie and I both had the sense that it wouldn't be the last signature.

Dana went in for the procedure at about 9:00 pm. Laurie was invited in. I was asked to wait in the waiting room. I have had some long hours in my life. Waiting for marks to come out during my undergraduate university years in mechanical engineering and trying out for rep hockey teams came to mind. That yearning feeling was brutal, as you waited for the professor to post the ranked grades, when I knew that I hadn't put in enough effort to receive a good grade or to even pass, but still somehow held out hope to move on. Or, the sickening feeling of skating in a circle around the ice with 40 other teenaged boys after a St. Albert Midget AAA hockey team tryout, watching the coach skate up to boy after boy, singling them out to cut them from the team.

Now I sat in a waiting room pining for the procedure to end and to hear the results, to know what the near future held for my daughter and my family. I hoped with all of my heart that Laurie and I were good parents and hadn't made some mistake at home that exposed Dana to the bug that was now hurting her. I hoped that the genes that we had passed on to her were strong enough; strong like they were when her own body attacked and destroyed her insulin-producing islet cells. I hoped for what I had no strong belief in. I hoped that God was with her. Then I waited some more.

The door swung open at a little after 10:00 pm. The team of doctors and nurses pushed Dana's bed through the hall and Laurie followed close behind. Laurie extended her hand out to me and I rose to my feet to join the procession winding its way through the hospital corridors.

"Do you think Dana's in trouble?" Laurie asked, clenching

my hand tightly. I paused for a second and then answered.

"Yes, I think she's in trouble!"

We didn't say another word as we followed the procession to yet another stopover room. Laurie and I sat down and Dana slept off the anesthetic. There was nothing to talk about, but my mind began to race. My next thoughts were abstractly connected to the scene. It dawned on me that Dana was receiving what had to be world-class care. I began to try to figure out what Laurie and I would have to pay for the team of professionals caring for Dana if it were out of our own pocket. I had been reading for years about extended waiting lists for MRI's and CAT scans. Dana had both within hours of coming to the hospital.

"Do you realize that Dana has had an MRI and a CAT scan in one day?" I asked Laurie, breaking the silence. "No waiting list!"

"Why the hell do you think that is? They don't get these tests because everything is fine, Jim." Laurie snapped. "Can we just wait for the results?"

"Yes. I guess so."

"Sorry," she whispered. "I'm tense and worried."

"It's alright. I didn't mean to upset you."

A new stranger walked through the door. We hadn't seen her yet. She introduced herself as a neurologist and as the person who would now oversee Dana's care. We hadn't been able to get any conclusive answers all day on what was actually going on with Dana. Hopefully they were coming now.

She explained the results of the CAT scan. Then she showed us the MRI results and how to look for the irregular shapes and formations on her left side as compared to the right side of her brain. It was unbearable to study the problems growing in Dana's head and my heart sank as the neurologist explained her diagnosis.

The bug had infected her mastoid bone behind her left ear and was destroying it. It had infected her left eardrum and the tiny hearing bones behind it. A blood vessel leading from her brain down the left side of her head, near the mastoid bone, was clotted and threatening to give her a debilitating or fatal stroke at any time. The bug had breached her skull and was releasing air, creating pockets of air between her menenges and her skull. The bug was gaining strength and Dana was losing it quickly.

"What's next?" Laurie asked.

"We're going to start Dana on an aggressive antibiotic drip," the neurologist confidently explained. "I call it the mother of all antibiotics. It seeks and destroys anything foreign to her body. It will attack the bug and start to kill it."

"Does she need surgery for this?" Laurie asked.

"That would be the worst-case scenario. We're going to monitor her progress on the antibiotics over night and give her another CAT scan in the morning."

"How long is Dana going to be staying in the hospital?" I pressed.

"I think that you had better plan on at least a few weeks of antibiotic therapy," she answered. "She's going to be here for a while to beat this one."

"We know that she's got a lower immune system because of her diabetes. Was her diabetes a factor in getting this bug?"

Laurie asked.

"I don't think so. I don't think so at all. They are most likely completely separate events."

"Is there something in our house or that we exposed her to that started this?" I asked.

"It doesn't work that way. The lab will find out what this bug is. You can rest assured that you didn't cause this just as surely as you didn't cause the diabetes."

"What do I do about sleeping arrangements?" Laurie jumped in.

"Oh, yes. They're going to set Dana up in the ward in the Stollery Children's Hospital here. You'll be set up in a parent's room."

"Could this kill Dana?" I asked, knowing the answer.

The neurologist leaned in, trying her best to pass her confidence and strength to Laurie and I. "I have seen this before at the Hospital for Sick Children in Toronto. I know what to do. We can save Dana. We're going to."

CHAPTER 10

Tuesday January 16, 2001

"Hello you guys! Dana and Rossco, where's Daddy's hug?" I announced walking into the driveway side door of our old bungalow.

"Me first! Me first!" Dana yelled, cutting Ross off and jumping into my arms.

Ross let out a frustrated whine and complained that it wasn't fair because Dana was bigger.

"You can get a hug too," I reassured Ross, dropping Dana on her feet and picking him up.

"How was your day?" Laurie asked, looking down at her plate, holding her head up with one hand and eating with the other.

"Chicken and French fries for dinner again?" I complained.

"I don't want to hear about it. I've had a hellish day," Laurie shot back.

Dana and Ross sat back at their seats on the bench at the kitchen table and continued with their dinner. "Were you sick again today?" I asked.

"I've been sick every day since getting pregnant with this rat. I don't know what I'm having, but this kid's nasty."

"July's coming," I reassured her and leaned in to whisper in her ear, rubbing my hands almost sarcastically, but still quietly hopeful. "I suppose getting a little tonight is out of the question?"

"Is that all you ever think about? Forget it. I'm sick! Talk to me in September, maybe."

I laughed, walked to the sink and poured myself a glass of water. Laurie's eyes lifted from her plate and her glare followed me.

"You've never been sick like this. Hell, you've never even had a headache," Laurie barked.

"I've had a headache before."

"Hangovers don't count!"

After placing my glass at my seat beside Laurie and making my plate up for dinner, I sat down with everyone and started to eat.

"What was her blood sugar?" I asked.

"It was eleven point two. We're going to need a new house you know?" Laurie stated, in between bites.

"Yes I know. We should have thought about that before making one too many kids for the number of bedrooms we have. Although, it seemed like a good idea at the time," I smirked.

Laurie grunted in disgust at my attempt at humour. "When should we start looking?"

I thought about the question for a moment, remembering

all the stories that my dad told me about life in Sudbury, Ontario when his family grew up stacked like fire wood in a tiny house, as he would put it.

"Dana and Ross are already sleeping in a room together. The baby can have the other room. We could wait a little while."

"Yes we could wait a little while, but Dana's getting older. How long do you think she's going to like having Ross in her room?"

"I don't know. We can't afford to do it now. We'll have to wait until we see what my bonus will look like this year. If we're going to sell, I'd like to put new siding and shingles on the garage and the house," I explained, while inhaling my supper.

"Why? To sell it?"

"Yes. But mostly to leave it a little better than it has been since we bought it. That poor old couple behind us keeps their house so nice and our garage siding is all dry rotted. I'm afraid that some young couple will buy our house like we did and not have any money to fix it up."

"Can we go skating?" Dana interrupted.

I looked at Laurie and she threw up her hands, leaving the decision to me.

"Where?" I asked.

"On the lake at Festival Place!"

"Alright."

"Yeah!" Dana cheered.

"I'll keep Rossco here, if that's alright," Laurie added.

"That's fine."

"Mommy. I'm done supper. Can I go watch TV?"

"Yes, Dana," Laurie answered, as Dana and Ross left the table and Laurie got up to clear their dishes. "Oh, Daddy, please give Dana her insulin."

"Not in the leg. Not in the leg!" Dana protested.

"The diabetes clinic called. We scheduled Dana's next appointment. Will you come with Dana and me again?" Laurie asked, while opening the dishwasher.

"Not this time. I think I'll just stay at work," I answered, getting up with my plate, taking it to the sink.

"Please put that in the dishwasher and not the sink. I'm not your cleaning lady you know!" Laurie complained. "It would be nice to have your support at the clinic."

I found Dana's insulin kit, sat back down at the table and measured the quick-acting and the long-acting insulin.

"I don't think you need my support there. You guys don't even acknowledge me at all."

"That's not true! I love that you're there," Laurie argued, sitting back down at the table across from me. "Do you want tea?"

"Come on! You and the nurses get talking, or the doctor, or the dietitian. Whenever I try to add anything you all look at me with that mock patient, uppity look, quickly and silently dismiss whatever I've said, and carry on," I clarified. "Sure I'll have some tea."

I motioned for Dana to come and sit on my knee. "Not here, Daddy!" Dana pleaded and she guided me to the couch in the living room.

"That's not how it is," Laurie tried to explain, as she stood up from the table and readied the orange pekoe tea.

"What do you mean that's not how it is? I just told you that's how it is," I said loudly from the living room as I gave Dana her shot.

"I'm sorry if you feel that way, but that's not what I'm trying to do. I honestly want you to come with me."

"Listen. You and the diabetes clinic have brushed off every idea that I've come up with."

"Jim, I'm the one that has to manage Dana's diabetes day in and day out. So you tried to come up with a few ideas and they didn't work," Laurie continued.

"What do you mean they didn't work? You didn't even give them a chance!"

"Statistical control charts, documenting everything Dana eats and the intensity of her activity levels, as well as her insulin shots and blood sugars, charting all these things, and whatever else you came up with, are all things that you do. I don't do those things! It's enough of a job for me to do the simple things like keep Dana alive every day."

"The kettle is boiling," I noted. "And that's not good enough. The last A-one-C blood sugar test that the nurse did was higher than her first. We don't have good control of her blood sugars. Her average blood sugar value is too high and the range of blood sugar levels between high and low during the day is too great."

"Why don't you quit your job and give it a try! Do you honesty think you can control this thing with statistics like some quality defect on your shop floor?" Laurie yelled.

I rubbed my eyes and pulled my hands over my face in

frustration. "This is crap!"

"What's crap? I have to be able to manage Dana's diabetes my way. It's my job. If you want it done differently, take the job, but I'm not trying to insult you by not following all of your ideas."

"Listen, do what you want, but I'm not coming to the next clinic appointment. You don't need me there at all," I barked, got up from the table, and left the room to gather the skates.

"Where are you going, Jim?"

"To get ready to go skating with Dana."

"Don't you want your tea?"

"No!"

Dana and I left for the skating rink on the lake by Festival Place. The temperature was a tolerable minus ten degrees Celsius, the air was still, and there were no clouds. I had a small pack with me to take onto the lake that included a few high carbohydrate snacks for Dana's extra activity, her glucometer, and an apple juice box just in case she went low.

We found a spot on the steps leading down to the manmade lake and set our gear down. I took out Dana's skates and removed her shoes.

"Not too tight, Daddy," she pleaded.

"Don't worry, Dana."

Once I'd finished tightening her skates and securing her helmet I tied up my own skates. I collected our gear and stored it on the raised bank, so that I could reach everything with my skates on. Then Dana and I were on the lake, skating laps, holding hands.

Hockey had been a central activity in my upbringing. My

father and older brother played at a high level and I had played on St. Albert's Bantam and Midget AAA teams during my teenage years. Any time I laced up my skates, it brought back memories. The smell of my well worn skates with my old number written on the bottom, the sting of the cold air piping through my nose following a few hard strides, the sound of ice flaking away under the strain of the metal blades during hard crossovers, or the simple feeling of the flesh on my fingers tearing slightly as I laced my skates properly were enough to make me feel at home.

Now, I was skating on the ice with my daughter. Dana was very different from me, more like her mother I suppose. She was tiny, but fearless. I could remember being scared of most new experiences when I was growing up. It took patience to get me to do something like skating or playing hockey. Once you got me into the activity, it took patience and methodical coaching to expand my abilities. However, those few coaches that understood how to move my shyness aside with the right kind of praise were pleasantly surprised by my growing abilities and desire. Dana needed no such coaching. She was willing to fall all night long, banging her hips, bum, elbows, and knees, only complaining for a moment when it really hurt. It was invigorating to be around her when her enthusiasm was splashed across her face and her tiny body exploded with untapped potential.

"Daddy, chase me!" Dana yelled.

"Daddy's coming to get you!" I growled, slowly skating behind Dana, pretending to pursue her as she squealed with delight at the fun.

I chased her around the lake for twenty minutes or so and played with her as she tried new things like skating backward or stopping.

"Come on, Dana. Let's get you something to eat for the activity."

We skated over to our gear and I rifled through the contents of the skate bag until I found the bag of snacks. I was still new at guessing how intense the activity was and how to balance what I was going to give her with how high her blood sugar was at supper. I reasoned with the simple rule that the diabetes clinic gave me during the summer, five carbohydrates for each twenty minutes of high intensity activity. I doled out the five-carbohydrate Arrowroot cookies using that formula. Dana ate them quickly and skated off again.

"Come on, Daddy!"

"Daddy's going to sit down on the steps for a few minutes. You go ahead and I'll watch you. Do some tricks for me."

I sat watching her skate and she checked in with me every few minutes to make sure that I was still watching her routines.

"Things look and sound much better than they did a few months ago," said an accented voice, from beside me. I turned to my left and looked at the face for a long moment before I recognized Father Wes.

"Hello again," I waved.

"It looks like you're having a great time with Dana tonight. Where's the rest of the family?"

"Oh, Rossco and Laurie stayed home tonight."

"How's Laurie's morning sickness going?"

"Lousy. Who told you she's pregnant?"

"People talk in this town. I hope she's feeling better soon."

"I hope so, too. What brings you here tonight?"

"I just came for a skate and to rest my mind from my work a little. You say I hope so too with some real feeling to it. Is something wrong?"

"Ah, Laurie and I had a bit of a fight tonight. Sometimes we argue about how to care for our kids, especially Dana. Laurie's so strong and unmovable in her opinions and that makes it hard at times."

"I suppose that you're really flexible," Father Wes commented with a smile on his face.

"I know, I know, I'm as stubborn as a mule, but it's hard for me when we're talking about the kids. I'm like a fish out of water on many of the issues. I'm at work all day and Laurie runs the show. I guess I'm not used to being the worker anymore. It bothers me not be the boss."

"What was the issue tonight, if you don't mind me asking?" Father Wes questioned, in a calm voice.

"I suppose I don't mind you asking. I was supposed to come see you anyway. We don't agree on how to manage Dana's diabetes. Laurie wants to only do a minimal amount of documentation and I would like to do more so that we can manage her disease with some data."

"That sounds like a lot of work for Laurie."

"Yes, but it would be useful information that could help Dana," I argued. "I put together the sheets for Laurie and I was going to do all of the data entry and graphing from the documentation that Laurie would record."

"Laurie doesn't like this idea. Correct?" Wes commented.

"What does like have to do with it? This is for Dana."

"Is it?" Father Wes asked.

"What?"

"Watch this, Daddy!" Dana yelled at me as she attempted to complete an awkward spin and fell flat on her bum.

"Great, honey! Keep it up," I encouraged.

"It appears to me that you're searching for a role in your daughter's diabetes. You want an active responsibility in her care, just like you want an active responsibility in your son's upbringing."

"Of course I do," I answered.

"Would you run your wife's day home to be close to Ross or would you prefer to engage him in physical activity?"

"I prefer to engage both Dana and Ross in physical activity. That's what I like to do."

"Excellent. And I bet Laurie doesn't like to do those things. She'd probably prefer to read to them and take them to museums. Right?" Wes continued.

"I guess so."

"Dana's diabetes is no different," Wes argued. "You need to find a leading responsibility that doesn't interfere with Laurie's leading responsibility too much. You are subordinate to Laurie's day to day care of Dana. Learn to be effective in that and find something else."

"But I'm so scared for Dana's future. I'm so scared that this disease is going to kill her before I'm ready for her to die. I just keep thinking that I need to be intimately involved with the disease so that I can help her," I argued.

Wes rubbed his chin and thought for a moment.

"I think you're searching for hope."

"Of course I'm searching for hope! I hope that diabetes is cured."

"There's only one place from which true hope can flow, and you need real faith to obtain this hope," Wes began.

"Wait a second," I interrupted as my defenses rose. "I know where you're going. I know that I have to find a way to get God back into my life, but curing diabetes is science."

Father Wes moved closer and put his hand on my shoulder.

"With what you know now about the disease, do you really think that curing diabetes would not be a miracle?"

"I suppose it could be interpreted that way."

"I'll take that for now," Wes smiled as he stood up to go skating. "Miracles are happening all around you, but it takes faith to see them. Search for your role in Dana's diabetes. Search for your faith and your hope will gain strength."

"I'll think about it, Father Wes," I answered as he skated away.

"Daddy, I'm hungry. Is it snack time?" Dana asked as she skated past Father Wes and up to me.

It was a little after 7:00 pm. Snack time was indeed getting close.

"I think you're right. Let's go home," I answered.

We arrived home just before snack time and Dana rushed to her room to put on her pajamas.

"I'm sorry about the fight," Laurie said as she gave me a hug.

"I'm sorry, too," I whispered.

"A lady named Joanne called tonight. She's from the

Alberta Foundation for Diabetes Research. She asked me to get you to call her back as soon as possible."

"I wonder what that's about?" I asked.

"I don't know. She told me that your boss, Don Oborowsky, got her to call."

CHAPTER 11

Saturday May 12, 2001

I couldn't sleep and had been catnapping at best all night. There was nothing that could make me sleep. That trusted and hated alarm clock of mine was set for 5:00 am. It was 4:30 am and I wouldn't need the alarm this morning. There was a vice-tight feeling in my stomach, the kind of feeling that I hadn't felt since my teenage years before important hockey games. My brother Steve would brew boiled coffee for me to get me wired and ready for important games, the kind of games where a tournament was on the line or a scout was coming to watch. I loved my brother, but the coffee really just made me want to puke.

In a weird way, this morning's anxiety was almost a welcome feeling, and although I felt tired there was an endurance building in me as the morning hours crawl by.

Dana's bedroom door was open and she was sound asleep. She was low last night, but she'd been fed and checked already. Just because there was nothing else to do I crept into her room and checked her blood sugar once more before her 8:00 am breakfast check. It read 9.6 mmol/l, which was in the good range.

The floor of our old bungalow creaked in all the same spots as I walked as softly as possible downstairs. The wet cedar aroma of the sauna my dad Ray and I built in my basement four years earlier still filled the air from last night's shower. I had set the temperature to 175 degrees Fahrenheit, which was perfect for me, and with the flip of the switch it was heating up again. The twenty-minute heat up period for the sauna gave me a little time to run out to my truck one more time to check on the gear that I had to bring to the track this morning. It was all there, just like it was last night when I checked it before going to bed.

Finally satisfied that I probably hadn't forgotten anything, I quietly walked back downstairs, stripped down, and entered the sauna. The bucket that my brother Steve and his wife Marilyn brought back from Costa Rica was filled with hot water from the tap below the shower head, and I threw a few heaping scoops onto the rocks after I settled onto the top bench. The white plumes of steam rocketed to the ceiling and then circulated the room, dousing my upper body in the soothing heat. Sweat was pouring out of me within minutes and I dumped more water onto the rocks. Fifteen minutes later, I had had enough steam and got down from the bench to turn on the shower. It was invigorating to have a cold shower in a hot sauna. The cold water slowly sprayed onto the hot rocks releasing even more steam. The moist heat totally surrounded you and penetrated deep into muscles.

Once I'd had my fill of shower and steam I opened the door to the bathroom and the door to the change-room to allow the moisture to escape. Then I found the little squeegee under the bench, wiped the walls and bench off, and directed the excess water on the drainage-flawed tile floor toward the drain.

I laid out all of my clothes for the day the night before, running shorts, running socks, the race shirt, a new track suit, and I put them on like a team uniform. I killed a little more time making myself a scrambled egg, ham, and cheese sandwich. By 6:00 am, it was time to go to the track. I'd made the decision last night to drink this day in, win or lose.

The sun was painting the low horizon with dim pinks and oranges as I pulled into the parking lot of the Strathcona Athletic Park in Sherwood Park. The access gates to the track were locked, but I had been furnished with keys for the event. Bill and Scotty showed up with the tents about five minutes after I arrived. We had just laid out the two 40 foot by 20 foot tents on the ground when Ray, Steve, and brother-in-laws Rob and Craig arrived. I hadn't expected this many volunteers so early, but it helped me to smile. Not long after that Laurie's brother and dad Al and Norm showed up to help set up the event and act as first aid doctors. We broke into teams and began the labour of erecting the two large tents on either side of the football bleachers.

"Good morning, you guys!" my boss Ted Degner yelled as he drove up a few minutes later.

He jumped out of the truck and joined the work. Before 7:30 am Joanne Langner, the Executive Director of the Alberta

Foundation for Diabetes Research, or AFDR, and her husband had shown up with a five-ton Mack truck full of tables, chairs, concession items, and signs for the race. Then my co-chairs for the race and the remainder of our committee appeared.

The site transformed into a bustling group of people directing the creation of various venues to generate the atmosphere we had designed for our first race. The two large tents were the focal point. The east tent would house the registration and the tent on the west side of the main north bleachers would house first aid and massage. There were two 12 person hot tubs set up beside the west tent and the concession shack was beside the east tent. A line of orange barricades marked off the baton exchange area on the eight-lane rubberized track in front of the bleachers.

"Where do we set up?" Laurie's cousin Kevin Fleming said as I spun to meet him.

"You made it! Awesome!" I exclaimed, reaching out to shake his hand.

"Made it? Hell yeah! Smokey Lake Alberta, pumpkin capital of the world, showed up with two junior high teams of ten, two high school teams of ten, and an entourage of support staff," Kevin added.

"That's great! You can set up anywhere in the rugby field west of the bleachers."

"Great! One more thing, we brought lots of money. Is that okay?" Kevin said, smiling.

"You're the best, pal!"

Other teams began to show up and the organizing committee members guided them to the registration tent.

Volunteers placed the event and sponsorship signs around the track. It wasn't a screaming success, but it was no failure for a first-year event that had only started to be pieced together in late January, a little over three months earlier.

Steve and Marilyn's team showed up and set up their tents. My friends from Waiward showed huge support by bringing over 50 participants. My smile inched bigger.

At approximately 9:20 am, a reporter from a Sherwood Park community newspaper showed up looking for me.

"Give me a little background about yourself and this event," he requested.

"My name is Jim Kanerva. I'm new to the Alberta Foundation for Diabetes Research Board of Directors and I'm co-chair of this event."

"What's the name of this event again?"

"It's the first annual AFDR 24-Hour Relay."

"What is the money being raised going toward?"

"All the money raised here is being used to fund the ongoing Type 1 diabetes research at the University of Alberta and the Islet Cell Transplantation Team. That's the team that developed the Edmonton Protocol."

"What's the Edmonton Protocol?"

"That's where they inject islet cells into a Type one diabetic's liver and stabilize the transplant with anti-rejection drugs. About eighty-five percent of the transplant recipients are still completely off insulin injections!"

"What does this mean to you?" the reporter asked, writing feverishly.

"It means that, from what Doctors Rajotte, Shapiro, Ryan,

and Lakey have told me there's a great chance that I'm going to see my daughter Dana cured, maybe before she's twenty!"

"Is that why you're out here?"

"Absolutely! The only thing holding these doctors back is money. That should be a simple problem to solve if enough people put their mind to it."

The reporter and I talked for a few more minutes as he gathered more in-depth information about the race, the Edmonton Protocol, and AFDR.

"Jim, come over here," Marilyn called from the registration tent. "We've got to discuss our team name."

"What are you thinking?" I asked, reaching the table.

"How about the Danasaurs?" she asked.

"Danasaurs?"

"Yes. The Danasaurs. Our team is all here because of Dana. Look at this, someone came up with the great idea of having these white stickers that we can attach to the shirts. The idea of the sticker is to write the name of the person you're running for on it."

I attached mine to my right chest, with Dana written in bold black ink on it.

"Jim, we've got a few problems," my co-chair explained as a crowd of family and friends gathered around her and me at about 9:30 am.

"What's up?" I asked.

"The breaker keeps blowing on the hot tub pumps. The Smokey Lake teams have set up a TV and other assorted electronic stuff on the same breaker. It just can't handle it."

"No problem," Ted Degner interrupted. "I'll head back to

Waiward and grab the diesel generator. We'll have you up and running within the hour."

"Perfect!" I said.

"Come on Ray," Ted urged, enticing my dad to go with him. "Let's go."

Another volunteer came over and told us that the registration tent was coming along fine. Everyone had registered, paid, and had received their long sleeved running shirts and baton. The concession was under control. The lap counting sheets were handed out. It was time to get things going.

"Everyone! It's time to begin," I announced over the loud speaker as runners from the 15 teams of ten began to assemble. "Please have your first runner on the track. They'll be running the first mile starting at ten am sharp."

George Laraque from the Edmonton Oilers showed up to help kick off the race and sign autographs, especially for the three junior high school teams. Sean Fleming, the kicker for the Edmonton Eskimos, and honourary Chairman of AFDR, was next at the mike to explain what AFDR did and the value of volunteerism. Before he could even start talking, my brother-in-law Al and Kevin Fleming, both long time Eskimo's season ticket holders, and the Smokey Lake kids serenaded Sean with the traditional salute following a successful Eskimo field goal: "You're the best! You always were the best! You'll always be the best!"

The crowd and Sean laughed. Of course, it could have been the other salute, which is yelled after Sean misses one: "You're the worst! You always were the worst! You'll always be the worst!"

Sean passed the mike to my co-chairs who spoke of their involvement and passion for the cause and thanked the crowd. This AFDR event, which used to be a five kilometer fun run, had been theirs for years. They had worked hard, but wanted it to grow. They were kind enough to let me bring my ideas to start a 24-hour relay to their committee and to help create this event, which had a much larger scale than they were planning and an aggressive plan for future growth.

Then it was my turn to speak. I briefly explained the format to the crowd. One person would be on the track running four laps of the 400-metre track and then would pass the baton to the next runner. Lap counters would count the laps and hand in the sheets to the registration tent, where team progress would be tracked and reported at designated intervals throughout the day and night.

Then, a volunteer brought me the up-to-date information from the registrations. Dana, Ross, and Laurie were now in the crowd. I began speaking again from the heart.

"I'm so happy to see many of my friends and family here supporting us. This race is a race that I grew up with in Sudbury, Ontario. My older sister Susan and I have talked off and on about putting something like this on since we were kids. Thank you for helping that little dream come true. Years from now, when this race is being run across Western Canada and raising big money for diabetes research, you'll have been here first to build it. This research is going to save my little girl Dana some day, and a lot of people like her. To help with that, all of you in this inaugural group of teams have raised $42,000 for the AFDR!" I announced, to the cheers of our modest crowd.

With that, George Laraque blew the air-horn sounding the start to our small event.

"Daddy! Daddy!" Dana came running over with Ross and very pregnant Laurie. "Is this my race?"

"Yes, Dana! This is your race. What do you think?" I asked her as I picked her up and hugged her.

"I have to run, too!" she announced, looking back at Mommy for permission.

"That's fine, Dana. How far are you going to run?" Laurie questioned.

Dana looked at the ground for a second and then ran her eyes around the track with the runners dispersed at various intervals.

"I am four years old. I will run four laps!"

"Dana, that's a long way. Are you sure that's how far you want to run?" I asked.

"Yes. Can we do it now?"

"No problem. Let me drop my stuff off at the tent and you and I will go," I answered.

Dana and I started her run at a slow pace, even for a four-year-old. However, to my surprise she began to run the laps away without changing her pace. As she finished her second lap the people around the track began to notice the tiny spectacle and cheered Dana on. It was fun to watch her warm to the encouragement being yelled to her from the strangers on the sideline. Her strides became stronger, her head lowered slightly, and she ran the last lap faster, appearing not to want to let her new fans down. The onlookers cheered as Dana crossed the finish line, completing a steady one-mile run. It was a quiet moment in the event that brought me great pride and drove the message home of why I was there.

"Is that as fast as you can run, old man?" Jeremy, a young coworker of mine chided as he slapped my back and watched Dana run from me to Laurie.

"I was just saving some up for you, punk," I shot back.

"When do you run?" he demanded.

"Whenever you want me to, young man."

"I'm next. I'll set the pace. Try to keep up," Jeremy laughed as he grabbed the baton from his teammate and ran off.

"Just remember you're a volleyball player, Jeremy," I yelled, watching him round the first corner.

"I'm timing him," my brother-in-law Al announced to the crowd of onlookers who had gathered to watch the fun.

As Marilyn came around to pass me the baton I looked for a timer.

"Steve, I'm gone. Time me."

"I got you," Steve called back.

"Jeremy's coming in for the first lap split," Al hammered it up. "It's, it's, it's one minute twenty two!"

"Jim's coming in for his red-hot split!" Steve called out to the growing crowd of hecklers. "He's through at, at, it's one minute seventeen! Holy crap, he's on fire!"

"You're going to have a heart attack, old man!" Al barked.

"Jeremy's coming in for lap two!" Al kept the suspense going. "He's by at about, it's, actually two minutes and forty eight seconds, dropping the pace a little."

"Jimmy's coming around to the straight-away," Steve jumped in. "Oh it looks fast! He coming by now, it's going to be, he's two minutes forty-one! Someone's shot his leg off!"

"You're fat and slow, old man!" Al laughed as I ran by.

"Split three! Split three!" Al yelled. "Jeremy is four minutes twenty one! He's dying a slow death here folks!"

"Jim's hopping around turn four!" Steve mocked. "That leg's getting tired now, but he's by at a snail's pace of, now it's four minutes and eighteen seconds! Still leading!"

"Bring it home, Jeremy!" Al yelled as the crowd cheered him on and doused him with a liberal dose of sarcastic comments. "And, he has crossed the line with a spirited time of five minutes and fifty two seconds, hardly a record of any kind!"

Jeremy caught his breath in time to curse me home, along with the small screaming crowd, having fun with the only runner on the fun run track running his ass off.

"Jimmer, bring it home you sorry idiot!" Steve encouraged. "And he's coming in, he's going to be through, he got a chance, he's through at, at five minutes forty seven seconds! It's a new race record!"

The day soon fell into a routine of lap running and the activities in between. The Smokey Lake gang set up a TV in their tent and we watched the NHL Playoffs, ate burgers, and laughed a bunch while telling old stories to each other. As the laps piled up, each team began to feel the effects of the mileage. The Danasaurs were turning laps at a steady pace and by the twelve hour mark I had run nine one-mile stints on a team of five women and five men. This was by no means a fast pace, but for recreational runners, it was grinding.

The daylight had faded away and the warm spring day had turned to a cool spring night. The teams were now quieted by the strain of the activity and the participants reflective of our accomplishments. By early morning, quiet rock music played from a boom box on a table in the east tent. Participants were now sleeping between four-lap runs. I loved this time of night and this event. Maybe this is why I wanted to put this on, just to feel this once. When Steve and Susan ran in the Sudbury 24-Hour Relay, they ran in the big event. I was in junior high school and was only allowed to run in the 12-Hour Relay. I had romanticized the 24-hour run for the rest of my adolescence.

I sat in the bleachers alone after my run between five and six in the morning. Flecks of daylight were appearing on the horizon. I hadn't slept all night. I felt great, but kind of road-stoned.

"So, what do you think?" Steve asked, sitting down beside me.

"About what?"

"About your event?"

"I think it's been good. I wish more people came out this year. I suppose this is a good turnout for how long we've been planning this."

"I think it's great! You've put on a good one, little brother."

I didn't answer. It felt good to hear that from someone I've spent my entire life trying to measure up to.

"Do you think that Dr. Rajotte and his doctors are going to get it done? Is the Edmonton Protocol the answer?" Steve asked.

"Yes and no." I answered.

"What do you mean?" Steve pressed.

"Doctor Rajotte says the transplant works, but you need too many donors to make a difference. Right now, two people have to die for Doctor Lakey to isolate enough islet cells for one transplant. Doctor Lakey's working on improving the isolation techniques so he'll only need one donor, but there are so many diabetics."

"What's the answer?" Steve asked.

"Doctor Rajotte thinks that the team can develop a procedure for using pig islet cells to transplant. Then there'd be an unlimited supply. When that happens, maybe Dana can get the transplant."

"She can't get it now?"

"The anti-rejection drugs apparently might cause worse side-effects in time than being Type one diabetic. Doctor Shapiro says that Dana is safer to stay as she is than risk a transplant now."

"Man, I hope the research gets you there, brother," Steve encouraged, slapping my back.

"That would be something wouldn't it? That's why I'm here. It would be unbelievable to be even a small part connected to curing Dana," I said, staring out at the coming dawn, tired, proud, and happy.

CHAPTER 12

Friday November 30, 2001

"Daddy!" Ross yelled as I swung open the door leading in from the garage of our new two-storey Sherwood Park home.

"Hey Rossco! How was your day?" I questioned after picking him up for a rough boy hug and dangling him upside down over my shoulder.

"Good," he replied once he was righted and on the ground.

"What did you do today, Rossco?" I questioned him, forcing him to stand still to talk to me for a few seconds.

"Um, ah, I played with Liam," he answered.

"Sounds like fun, pal," I said while ruffling his hair and sending him back to the kitchen to hang around Laurie's leg.

"Daddy! My turn!" Dana barged into the back entrance.

"Come give me a hug! How was your day?" I asked.

"It was good. I went to play school."

"Where's your baby brother, Eric?"

"He's napping."

"What else happened today?" I asked.

"Um, I got into trouble," Dana responded and lowered her head once she had finished.

"Trouble? What kind of trouble?" I demanded.

"Jim, you've got to go to the store and pick up something to cook tonight," Laurie pleaded. "Leah and Avery are coming over for dinner. They'll be here by seven."

Leah is my cousin, is the same age as me, and is a great friend. She's an elementary school teacher and her husband Avery, also a great friend, is an actuarial accountant. He's an unbelievable mathematician; sets crop insurance rates in Alberta, and is starting to gain attention for his talents around the world. Who knew actuarial accounting could be so exciting?

Even more peculiar is the fact that Avery is a fun guy to be with. Not that I should be talking too much with my engineering background.

"Alright, I'll go pick up some groceries," I answered. "What happened to Dana today?"

"I'll tell you about it when you get back from shopping," Laurie explained, turning to go back to the kitchen. "Don't worry about the kids I'll feed them while you're gone."

"Okay," I answered, grabbed my keys, and went to the grocery store.

Cooking special dinners was always my role since Laurie and I started going out more than 13 years ago. She didn't like the added stress of cooking for guests. My mom, on the other hand, had spent numerous hours with me in her kitchen when I was a boy. She taught me how to make breakfasts, then some simple baking like cookies and cakes, and finally full meals. I developed a love for it and took it from there. Tonight, I'd keep things simple for myself due to the tight time constraints, but still have some fun in the kitchen.

We'd been in our new home for one week now. One of the complaints that I had about our old home was that I couldn't visit with the guests in the living room when I cooked. I finally knocked the walls down to make the dining room, living room, and kitchen into a sort of great room. When I went out shopping for a new home I had a few improvements that were mandatory. There had to be an attached two-car garage, two floors with four bedrooms upstairs, and finally a great room with a large kitchen. Laurie and I lucked out and found our new home, complete with my wish list items, in a quiet cul-de-sac.

Tonight I'd mess up that new kitchen making homemade linguini with Italian sausage tomato sauce.

"Honey, I'm home again!" I shouted as I walked into the house for the second time.

"What are you making?" she asked.

"Pasta and sauce."

"What did you get for dessert?"

"I bought a fresh pineapple."

"What? That's not dessert. Where's the chocolate?" Laurie complained.

"We don't need chocolate. Fresh fruit is a good dessert."

"Leah and I are going to have to go to Tim Horton's now and get some coffee."

"You're addicted to that stuff, you know. It'll kill you," I teased her while sorting out the groceries in the kitchen.

"Whatever. How many bottles of wine did you buy?"

"A red and a white."

"And you're not addicted to that stuff?"

"It's medicinal. There's heart disease in my family."

I pulled a large Dutch oven out from the island cupboard and set it on the stove. Then I cooked the mild Italian sausage in the microwave until firm enough to slice and put into the pot to brown. Next I added the onion, garlic, carrots, and green peppers into the pot with the fresh basil and parsley. Finally, I mixed in a good shake of Montreal steak spice, lemon juice, and Worcestershire sauce and then the diced tomatoes. After seasoning the sauce with the salt and spices, and letting it simmer for a few hours, about 30 minutes before we ate I'd add the diced asparagus.

After the sauce was left simmering, it was time to get at the pasta. I'd tried a few recipes over the years and had settled on a simple one that I could remember without looking it up each time. I added olive oil, eggs, durum semolina, all-purpose baking flour, garlic, salt, and basil together in a bowl. Then the mixture was tinkered with, mixed and kneaded until it had the feel that I knew would go through the pasta maker. I made enough to ensure leftovers, which was a must in my mother's kitchen. Once kneaded, the dough balls were set under a damp cloth to rest for twenty minutes. I'd opened a bottle of wine at the start, and had sipped my way through a glass by now.

"Someone's here!" Dana yelled after the doorbell rang.

"Can you answer that, Lo? I've got pasta all over my fingers right now."

Laurie, Dana, Ross, and Sasha met Leah and Avery at the

front door.

"Homemade pasta! Awesome!" Leah exclaimed upon entering the kitchen with her own bag of goodies. "What's for dessert?"

"Fresh fruit," I answered, proud of myself.

"I knew it. Ave, you owe me," Leah laughed as she bent down and picked up Eric to hold him for a while.

"Could you be a little less predictable, Jim?" Avery complained, stuffing two more wine bottles on the table and putting another bottle of something in the freezer.

"Fresh fruit is healthy. Speaking of healthy, with the amount of booze that the two of us have bought it looks like it's going to be one of those nights," I noted, while running the dough through the pasta maker, making short lengths of thick linguini.

"Ave's been in Chile doing crop stuff and he's got a surprise for you after dinner, Jimbo," Leah kidded.

"Oh, it's awesome stuff. The Chileans are crazy about it!" Avery chimed in.

"How old is Eric now?" Leah questioned. "He's huge already!"

"Isn't he ridiculous?" Laurie complained. "He's just about twenty weeks."

"At least he lets me hold him. He's so content. Dana and Rossco wouldn't let me near them as babies. Eric loves when Daddy holds him," I beamed.

"He lets anyone hold him," Laurie teased.

"Thanks," I sneered, going back to finishing the pasta and arranging it on wax paper on a cookie sheet.

"It's snack time, Dana and Ross!" Laurie announced, drawing the kids attention away from Dora the Explorer on the television.

They came running to the kitchen, took one look at the fresh pineapple and begged for slices.

"At least someone appreciates your dessert," Leah remarked, as I cut twenty carbohydrates worth of pineapple for each kid. Dana worked with Laurie to finish her blood sugar reading.

"Perfect reading, Dana! It's nine point three," Laurie announced.

"She sure is a good kid," Avery commented.

"And tough," Leah added.

"Oh, yeah! What happened to Dana at school today?" I asked, remembering the earlier broken conversation.

Dana's head sunk again. "Do you want to tell Daddy, Dana? It's alright," Laurie encouraged.

Dana simply shook her head refusing. "Dana was acting up in play school today. Her teacher asked Dana to stop whatever she was doing and Dana told her she was low," Laurie explained.

"What happened next?" I pressed, pouring water, salt, and olive oil into the large stockpot and putting it on the heat to boil.

"Dana asked to have her blood sugar tested and the teacher didn't do it."

"You're kidding?" I questioned, turning my head from the stove as Leah and Avery began to pay closer attention to the conversation.

"Unfortunately, I'm not. I don't know what I should do

about this situation," Laurie continued.

I shook my head. "She is the most caring teacher I've ever met. She loves Dana! What happened here?"

"I don't know. I think she thought that Dana was trying to manipulate the situation by using her diabetes as an excuse for acting up," Laurie reasoned.

"I want diabetes!" Ross yelled, pushing his plate of sliced pineapple hard across the kitchen table.

The adults stopped talking for a moment to consider Ross's announcement. I looked to Laurie to talk to him and she at me.

"Why do you want diabetes, Ross?" Laurie asked him.

"I want to be like Dana!" he demanded, grabbing her glucometer case.

"Do you want Daddy to do your blood sugar to see if you are diabetic?" I asked, looking to Laurie for reassurance, as Leah and Avery looked on silently.

"Yes!" he responded, holding his right thumb out, as Laurie put her hand to her mouth.

"Okay, Rossco. This will pinch a little," I explained as I pricked his thumb with the lancet and squeezed it for blood.

Ross jerked his hand as the lancet gouged his thumb and Dana looked on curious to see the result. I dipped the glucometer strip into the drop of blood forming on Ross's thumb and then we waited for the countdown to end.

"There, Rossco. Your blood sugar is five point three. Perfect!"

"See, Ross. You're not diabetic. Only I am," Dana soothed him and rubbed his shoulder.

Ross did not look satisfied with the result. Laurie had paid close attention to the proceedings and decided to soothe Ross a little further.

"Ross, I know we sometimes pay more attention to Dana than to you. Daddy and I love you the same. Dana has diabetes and we need to watch it closely or she could become very sick. I hope you can understand that."

Ross shook his head yes, but didn't say anymore.

"How would you like it if Daddy told you a Mako and Jet story tonight before bed?" I asked.

"Yeah!" Dana and Ross exclaimed.

"Okay then, it'll be Rossco's choice. You guys run upstairs, put on your pajamas, brush your teeth, and I'll come up and tell you a story."

"It's dark upstairs, Daddy," Ross complained. "You come with me."

"Rossco, you're perfectly safe. There's nothing to be afraid of in the dark. Turn on the light in your room when you get up there," I reassured him.

"No. You come with me."

"Dana, will you go with Ross and turn on his light so he's not scared?" I asked, shaking my head at Ross's intense fear of the dark.

"Yes, Daddy."

Laurie smiled a thank you and poured herself a glass of wine. Laurie usually read the kids one bedtime story each every night before tucking them in. I relieved her once in a while, but I wanted my turns to be different from hers sometimes. I invented stories for them that I would tell without a book, with only the nightlight on, while they cuddled me close. They

hung on every word that would come out, even if I struggled
with a story line on the spot. Over time, one set of characters
excited them more than others and it became a serial story.
The idea of a good orca named Jet patrolling the oceans, saving
unsuspecting victims from Mako the evil shark and his wicked
friends caught Dana and Ross's imagination.

Tonight's episode had Mako threatening Flounder and the
other peaceful residents of Vancouver's English Bay until Jet
came in to save them.

"Okay, Rossco and Dana, it's time for bed," I announced
after Mako had been chased out of English Bay's Kelp Reef
Manor once and for all.

"Juice and cheese!" Ross demanded.

Dana and Ross got into their beds and I prepared their cups
of Crystal Lite and a piece of sliced cheese. I brought Ross his
and then Dana.

"Sasha, Daddy?" Dana asked.

"You get up and call her to your bed, Dana. She's your dog,"
I coached.

"Okay," She answered, getting up from her bed. Dana then
walked to the top of the stairs and called the dog.

She smiled as the scraping sound of Sasha's claws could
be heard dragging across the kitchen floor as Sasha slowly
came to her friend's call. While I was putting the other kids
to bed, Laurie had tucked little Eric into his crib for the night
with a clean diaper after he'd finished yet another of the day's
numerous bottles. Then Laurie and I descended the stairs back
to our waiting guests.

"Sorry about that," I apologized.

"Not at all," Avery responded, as he tinkered with our computer.

"Let's get some dinner into us!" I announced, adding the pasta to boiling water.

I loaded each of the four plates with a generous portion of the fresh pasta and Italian sausage tomato sauce, and topped it with some fresh grated Parmesan cheese. Laurie and Leah prepared the salad that Leah and Avery had brought and Laurie opened and poured some more wine. Once we were seated at the table, the four of us smiled and drew in a collective breath of relief.

"Here's to sleeping kids," Laurie toasted and we joined her.

"How do you like the new house so far?" Avery inquired.

"Oh, it's been fantastic! But, I wish we could get everything unpacked," Laurie commented.

"I know what you mean, we've been in our new home for more than two years and I still don't have everything unpacked," Leah laughed.

"How's the teaching going this year?" I asked Leah.

"It's going great, but I don't want to get into an argument about the teachers' union, or teachers' anything with you tonight. Especially with the way you and Avery will be in a little while," Leah noted.

"Alright then, please pass the white wine, Ave," I laughed.

"Hey what did you guys do for Dana's Halloween?" Avery questioned.

"Do you mean all the candy?" Laurie responded.

"Exactly, how do you handle those kinds of situations?" Leah questioned. "I've wondered about that with Dana."

"Lo's actually the one who came up with that," I said, looking at Laurie to continue with the explanation.

"Oh, well for Halloween, Dana and I go through a little list of small things she wants, like Disney videos. I buy a few and she gets to buy them from me using her Halloween candy as money. In that way she can enjoy the experience of trick or treating even though she can't eat all of the candy."

"She still gets to eat some of the candy?" Avery questioned.

"Yes. She gets to eat some, but not as much as I let Ross eat. She gets a little for treats here and there. The problem is that every carbohydrate she eats as candy is one that she can't eat for healthy things. So, I keep it to a minimum," Laurie explained.

"That's a neat trick. I wouldn't have thought of that," Leah added.

"The pasta's excellent, Jim!" Avery complimented, with Leah and Laurie joining him.

"Thank you! It's nice to have you guys over. We don't get together nearly enough," I said.

"Hey, how did the race go this year?" Leah asked.

"It was a great time. We brought in about forty-two thousand," I answered.

"Are you doing it again?" Avery asked.

"Yes. Plans for next year are already under way. I've got a committee set up and I've already got over twenty thousand in corporate sponsorships!" I announced.

"When is it again?" Laurie jumped in.

"It's on May 4, 2002."

"Who's sponsoring?" Leah asked. "Any names we'd know?"

"The Cosmopolitan Clubs have collectively sponsored me

for over thirteen thousand. That's three times what they did this year!" I explained.

"Sounds neat. And all this is going to the doctors at the U of A that are doing the Edmonton Protocol?" Avery asked.

"Every penny!" I answered with pride. "Like I say, those guys are going to save Dana. They're close. They do more transplants every month and the program is going worldwide now. The US Federal Government gave ten million dollars and other major sponsors are coming on board. They're also very close to having the transplants fully funded by Alberta Health Care."

Laurie sighed. "Jim gets all pumped up every time he goes to an AFDR Board meeting or to one of his run committee meetings," she explained. "He comes home jacked up like a kid."

"It must be nice to be part of something like that," Leah stated.

"It's the best. It makes it worth getting up each morning," I added.

"Hey, I need something for dessert, and pineapple isn't going to cut it. Why don't you and Avery clean up while Leah and I go to Tim's for some coffee," Laurie suggested.

"Sounds great!" Leah agreed.

"I think it sucks!" Avery grunted.

The girls ignored any protesting that we attempted, put on their winter gear and disappeared walking down the bike path to the Tim Horton's less than two blocks away. I started the cleanup of the dinner dishes after slicing up the remainder of the pineapple for Avery and I. Avery dug into the freezer and pulled out a brown paper bag.

"What the hell is that?" I asked.

"Pisco! It's Chilean brandy," Avery answered. "I'm making you a Pisco sour. The Chileans got me stupid on this stuff one night down there."

Avery prepared the lime juice, Pisco, icing sugar, and crushed ice while I completed the dishes. I wasn't paying attention to the mixture he was putting together. After completing the cleanup of the dishes and the wine bottles, I sat at the table and devoured another slice of pineapple.

"Here, try this," Avery encouraged, handing me the green icy drink.

"Wow! It's good!" I exclaimed.

"No doubt, man!" Avery agreed, after we'd both taken large slurps of the drinks.

"Are you still doing those control charts for Dana?" Avery asked.

"Oh, yeah. I compile all of Dana's blood sugars, her insulin injection data, and how many lows and highs she's had. I put it all together for her letter that I give her on her birthday every year."

"You mean the one that she can't open until she's twenty one?" Avery asked.

"Yes, that's the one," I continued. "I take the blood sugar readings and I put them into a control chart for her. The X-Bar control charts show her average blood sugar reading, the upper control limit blood sugar value, and the lower control limit blood sugar value. The R-Bar chart shows the average range of her blood sugar readings, the upper control limit range, and the lower control limit range."

"How does the blood sugar data look graphically? Are you in control?" Avery asked.

I took another long pull from the Pisco before answering. "It's the worst. If it was my job I'd be fired! The average is fine, but the average range is like ten or eleven every day!"

"What do your pals the researchers say about that?" Avery asked.

"I haven't told them too many specifics about Dana, but every presentation that Doctor Shapiro makes focuses on the devastating effects that huge ranges in blood sugar levels have on a diabetic's body. That's what will slowly kill her."

"How's Laurie doing with everything?" Avery questioned.

"She's awesome. She's having a little bit of a rough week this week. She forgot to give Dana her insulin on Wednesday and had to go to playschool to give her the shot. She thinks she's a bad mother when stuff like that happens."

"My God, man, I don't know why she'd think that. Anyone could make those mistakes," Avery added.

"Oh exactly. I think Lo is questioning how her anti-depressants are working right now. It's pretty awesome how she handles everything with our family, and still has to deal with her own medical condition. I tried to tell her that her troubles this week are just the stress of the move, but she's got to work these things out for herself, I guess," I finished, and drank the last of the Pisco.

"Another Pisco it is then!" Avery announced, standing up from the table as he chugged the last of his drink down.

Avery mixed another two Pisco sours, handed me one, and

then went to the computer. He pulled up one of the free music sites and we selected a few songs that were good to laugh and sing to. We sipped at the new Piscos and exercised our sorry excuses for voices on such memorable tunes as Willie Nelson's "Poncho and Lefty", George Strait's "I've Come to Expect It from You", U2's "New Year's Day", and Billy Joel's "Only the Good Die Young".

"Hey, this stuff is pure booze!" I finally yelled to Avery over the music.

"You're just noticing now?" he laughed and grabbed my empty glass and finished his own. "Another Pisco it is then my good man!"

Avery went back to the kitchen and laboured over the increasingly difficult procedure of following his own recipe for the drink.

"Hey you two drunks, turn the music down!" Leah yelled as she and Laurie walked into the kitchen.

"Fine, fine, don't get angry," I answered, turning the volume down. "However, you know this means Avery and I are going to have to kick your ass at some game now."

"Oh, great! I love playing a game with Jim when he's drunk," Leah complained, watching Avery hand me another Pisco.

"It'll be different this time, I promise!" I responded, only to receive a disbelieving sneer from Leah.

Laurie and Leah finally agreed to a game of hearts. We set ourselves up at the kitchen table and dealt the cards, with the boys being aggressive and loud, as usual. Five hands into the game Laurie and Avery began to create some space between the bloated scores that Leah and I were racking up. Avery was winning with the lowest score. "Leah, what the hell are you doing?" I demanded, as she sloughed the queen of spades on me again instead of waiting to give it to Avery or Laurie. "I'm getting blown out of the water."

"Quit your whining. You don't know what's in my hand do you?" she snapped back.

"I'm surrounded by amateurs, man!" I complained, throwing my arms in the air.

"You're the one who's losing, honey," Laurie added.

"Hey, so what are you guys going to do about Dana's teacher?" Avery asked.

"Nothing, I guess. If a teacher as great as she is can make this mistake, then anyone can," I explained.

"I'm a teacher and I think it's kind of scary to even have that responsibility," Leah said. "It would crush me if I ever missed anything and a kid like Dana got hurt because of it. We don't receive any Type one diabetes training."

"I know what you're saying. I've come to the conclusion that Dana's got to be able to manage her diabetes independently," Laurie said. "That's why we held her back so she'll be the oldest in the class versus the youngest with a January second birthday."

"I think what she's got to do next time is tell the teacher that she needs her blood sugar done. If the teacher won't do it, Dana will," I added.

"Do you think that Dana was using diabetes to manipulate a situation where she was doing something the teacher didn't like?" Avery questioned.

"Ave!" Leah snapped.

"No, no, it's a fair question," Laurie defended him. "She says that she wasn't, but she might have been. However, the teacher has to prioritize what to do. If Dana says she needs her blood sugar tested the teacher should test it. If it ends up being normal too many times, then the teacher can start to deal with the manipulation factor and I'll support her. Just do the blood sugar first."

"I agree with my wife on this one," I seconded.

"What a tough position to be in for Dana and the teacher," Leah sighed.

"I know. I worry about her every day," Laurie agreed. "She goes to half-day kindergarten next year and then full-time grade one in 2003."

"It's your lead, Laurie," Avery urged as we started another round of hearts.

"Are you guys doing the flu shot thing again this year?" Leah questioned.

"Without a doubt!" Laurie exclaimed. "I hate it when Dana gets the flu. I don't sleep."

"I get the shot at work every year now," I explained. "I don't need another round of Dana having the flu again like she did a few months after being diagnosed. When Rossco gets it, it's bad enough, but once was enough with Dana."

The card game ended with the wrong person winning, which is anyone but me. Of course, I verbally abused everyone for allowing Avery to win and not playing smarter. Of course, they accepted none of my abuse and were more than happy to send some verbal jabs my way.

"Ave, I think it's time to go," Leah quietly instructed.

"What! We need one more Pisco," Avery objected.

"Absolutely! What would the evening be without one final Pisco toast?" I announced.

"No!" Leah and Laurie countered, sending Avery scurrying for the door and me following close behind.

"Good night you guys!" Laurie and I sent them off. "It was great to see you."

"Thanks! The dinner was great, your new home is beautiful, the singing sucked, and Jim wasn't too obnoxious at cards," Leah teased and Avery simply waved as he stumbled down the driveway.

"I'm tired and going to bed," Laurie announced after closing the front door. "Are you coming?"

"I'm going to stay up and watch a movie for a little while," I answered.

"Good night you drunken bum. I love you," Laurie yawned.

"I love you too. Good night."

There was an old Eastwood western that I found while flipping channels on the new flat screen TV we'd bought for the big space above the gas fireplace. I lay down on the couch and got into the movie. Before long I was dozing off and decided to wander up to bed.

When I reached my side of the bed, Laurie had laid Dana's glucometer on my pillow, as had become her custom. She was becoming even more adept at managing Dana's diabetes and was comfortable enough to give me some ongoing responsibilities. I picked up the case and quietly wandered into Dana's room. Sasha was sleeping on Dana's bed, woke, and wagged her tail. Dana had become used to this process and didn't wake easily during the finger prick and squeeze. She barely opened her eyes to eat if I had to treat a low in the night. The reading was good this time, but not great at 7.5 mmol/l. I had to treat anything lower than this number to give her enough energy to last through the night. I decided that she didn't need any food because she wasn't that active tonight and we didn't give her a big dose of long-acting insulin. After tucking her back under her covers, I went to bed, ready for it, and didn't set the alarm to check Dana again.

"Did you hear that?" Laurie forcefully whispered, knocking me in the side, waking me from a deep sleep.

"What? What time is it?" I yawned, straining my eyes to see my hated clock. "God, Lo, it's three thirty!"

"I think the dog barked," she continued.

"It was probably me snoring. Go back to sleep."

"No. Something's wrong. Go check where the dog is," Laurie begged.

"Laurie!"

"Jim, please!" she begged.

"Fine, fine, I'm going," I answered, crawling out of bed wondering why I was wasting my time.

Sasha usually barks in the middle of the night if she has to go outside to urinate so I checked the back door downstairs. She wasn't there. I walked around the house whispering her name, but she didn't answer. I finally came back upstairs and checked the kids' rooms. Sasha was sitting up on Dana's bed looking at me, very awake. She never remained in Dana's room after Dana fell asleep, preferring to be in our room or downstairs by herself. I looked at her for a second, thought about the situation, and returned to my bed.

"Where's the dog?" Laurie questioned.

"She's on Dana's bed," I answered, laying back down and tucking myself in.

"I'm going to check her blood sugar. Sasha never stays on Dana's bed this long," Laurie said.

"Fine."

Laurie was gone long enough for me to start falling asleep again.

"Jim! Wake up!" Laurie commanded, sitting down on her side of the bed. "Look at the reading."

She showed the glucometer reading she'd just taken. It was 1.6 mmol/l, which meant Dana was only several minutes to possibly an hour away from completely crashing, depending on how fast her blood sugar was dropping. In either case, with her parents asleep, Dana would have been in imminent peril. Laurie left the room, treated Dana's low with juice, and returned to bed.

"This scares the shit out of me!" Laurie whispered, with tears forming in her eyes. "What if I hadn't got up?"

"I don't know. Maybe it would be like your dad always says, her liver would purge the stored glucose and she'd wake up high."

"How many times can her body do that before it loses its ability to? What if one night it can't do that at all? What damage does it do to her when it does do that, if it even can?" Laurie cried.

"I don't know, Lo. I'm sorry I didn't feed her."

"It's not you. The last reading is fine. I would have done the same thing," Laurie reassured me. "What woke me up?"

"Didn't you say the dog barked?"

"Did it bark or did I dream it barked?" Laurie questioned.

"What do you mean?"

"Do you think God is looking out for Dana and is helping us?" Laurie wondered, wiping the tears from her eyes and regaining her composure.

"The dog was up. Maybe she's got a connection with Dana. She's spent a lot of time with that kid. You've seen some of those TV shows where dogs can even sense when their owners are going to have a seizure," I reasoned.

"God, I hope she can. I would just die if we lost her to a night-time low," Laurie stated. "Please set your alarm for five thirty and I'll check her again."

"Okay. Are you alright?"

"I'll be fine in the morning," she answered.

CHAPTER 13

Wednesday June 12, 2002

"Lo?" I yelled swinging the garage door recklessly open into the laundry room. "Are you packed and ready to go yet?"

I could tell that Laurie and her mom Marg had spent the early morning cleaning the house while I was at work. There was a fresh scent of Mr. Clean in the air and the kids' toys weren't haphazardly strewn around the living room as they normally were. Marg was staying at our house until Friday, helping us out again, as was normal for both Laurie's and my parents. June was the fun time of the year for kindergarten and playschool so the kids didn't want to miss out on anything. Marg was taking care of Ross and Dana at our house so that they could go to school and then she was taking them to St. Albert for the weekend where they could swim until they were sick of it. Laurie and I would drop Eric off at my mom's on our way to the airport.

"I'm packed, but I'm not ready. I'm not sure I'm ready at all," Laurie yelled down from our bedroom.

"It's too late for that now!" Marg pointed out from the kitchen, where she was putting the finishing touches on the morning dishes.

It may not be the most exiting trip to be going on, but it was a trip. We hadn't been on a trip together without the kids since Dana was diagnosed in July 2000. This was a working trip, but there would be plenty of opportunities for vacation activities. The Canadian Institute of Steel Construction Annual General Meeting was in Halifax this year. My employer, Waiward Steel Fabricators was a significant member company in this organization. I was the Presiding Officer of the Alberta Provincial Occupational Committee for the Alberta Steel Detailer Certificate Program. Instead of coming up with a shorter name, our committee was in the midst of an aggressive implementation of an Alberta Provincial Government certified drafting apprenticeship program. I had been asked to come to Halifax to deliver an update speech to the National Committee on Steel Detailing. This committee was interested in implementing our work on a national scale. In addition, my capstone project for my master's degree had been to set up a benchmarking network for the Canadian Institute of Steel Construction Member Fabricators. The 40 or so participating members paid me $250 per year each to do this study and I donated the money to the Alberta Foundation for Diabetes Research. I was delivering a speech on this ongoing work, as well. What that mundane agenda had bloomed into was a trip to a beautiful city for the price of a few hours work preparing and delivering two presentations.

Laurie struggled down the stairs with her suitcase, placed it in the front entrance by Eric's gear, and went to the kitchen to prepare a cup of tea for Marg and her. Eric was busying himself in front of the TV with a Scooby Doo video. Dana and Ross were still at school. Laurie had said her goodbyes to them at breakfast. I had gone to work early to finish with a few items needing attention. I bounded up the stairs with my laptop to pack my suit bag and ensure that my laptop bag had all of my work needs for the presentations.

I'm not sure when I actually developed the habit of leaving all of my packing for a trip to less than one hour before I was to depart. I had always done this during my hockey tournament years, but had never shown up to a tournament game having made the dreaded mistake of leaving my athletic supporter at home. The habit did add some stress, but by this time in my life it was more of a highly controlled stress. One positive side effect was that my luggage was usually considerably less voluminous than Laurie's.

Once I'd finished quickly stuffing suits, casuals, shorts, and the remainder of my travel needs into my computer bag and suit bag I checked the travel itinerary in the binder I'd prepared for the trip. My trip binder made Laurie laugh. It was one of the things that I did that screamed to the world that I was an engineer. Everything was in good shape and I was ready to go. I grabbed my bags, descended the stairs, and dropped my bags in front of Laurie's and Eric's. "Is this all that you're bringing, Lo?"

"Yes, that's everything."

"Are you sure you've got it all? Do you want to check?" Marg quizzed.

"It's all there, Mom," Laurie responded.

"Can I load this stuff into my truck or not?" I demanded.

"Yes, go ahead already," Laurie shot back.

"Are you alright?" Marg asked Laurie out loud.

"Mom!" Laurie exclaimed, heaving her hands forward, palms up, begging for an end to the discussion.

I let Sasha into the back yard so she wouldn't run away while I left the front door open to load the truck. We were never quite able to train her to stop running away. One of the daily torments that Laurie had to deal with was an absent-minded child leaving the door open for a few seconds while entering or leaving the house. Sasha was quick and always on the lookout for an opportunity to run. However, she never went very far once she'd escaped the house. It was almost like a game to her, just to see if she could do it. It was a good thing the dog had so many great qualities or Laurie would have made me get rid of her already.

Once the truck was packed I went back into the house to coerce Laurie to leave Marg in charge and come with me to Halifax. I found her at the kitchen table with Marg. Laurie was completing her briefing of the written instructions she'd left for Marg to care for Dana. "Is everything clear, Mom?" Laurie asked. "Do you have any questions before I go?"

"No. I think you've pretty much covered everything I need to know. You just go and enjoy some rest away from everything here," Marg answered.

"Are you sure, Mom?" Laurie prodded. "Everything's clear?"

I interrupted, "Laurie, you're mom's pretty smart. She'll be able to handle anything that comes up. We should be going already."

"I know, I know," Laurie answered, circling the room, looking for who knows what and holding her hand to her forehead. "Just follow the instructions Mom and you'll be fine."

"Lo! Come on, it'll be okay," I encouraged her.

Laurie finally made her way to the front entrance, put on her shoes, and walked out the door leaving Marg in charge. I picked up Eric, let him give Marg a goodbye hug, and put his shoes on. "Have fun, you two!" Marg called out just before we closed the truck doors and pulled away from the driveway.

Laurie was quiet and appeared uneasy all the way to St. Albert, where we dropped Eric off with my mom. The silence continued to the airport and I didn't try to overcome it with any small talk. I didn't feel as she felt. I was not in charge of Dana's care, responsible to manage the weight of the daily vigil that is ensuring the health of a Type 1 diabetic. I'm merely an employee in this case. I get to escape to work every day, thereby lessening the strain on me from caring for Dana. There was no escape for Laurie, day or night, until today.

We completed all of the required tasks at the airport and eventually boarded the jet, an Air Canada Airbus. The jet wasn't full so we were lucky enough to have a spare seat to allow us to stretch out a bit. Laurie said little and looked worried, possibly even a little paler now. To top things off, she hated planes too. Even the slightest bit of turbulence felt unnatural to her and caused her anxiety to heighten. The jet taxied and then roared to life, the wings slicing through the air, lifting us eastward into the deep blue Alberta sky. Laurie gripped my hand tightly, which allowed the heat of her worry to form a layer of sweat between both our palms. Her grip remained constant and strong while she concentrated on a Terry Brooks novel that she produced from her carry-on before we taxied down the runway.

A few minutes later, the jet leveled off and the flight attendants commenced with their regular service routines. Laurie let go of my hand, drew a deep breath, and sighed. She looked up from her book and turned toward me. A smile grew on her face. It was a gentle and enticing smile, the kind that coaxes you to smile back without you even realizing it. She undid her seat belt and moved toward me. I extended my hand to her. She took it, wrapped her other arm around my neck, and gave me a brief kiss on my lips. "Thank you. This is going to be a wonderful trip," She whispered in my ear.

"I'm happy you came," I whispered back.

Laurie patted my thigh and moved back to her seat. Colour had returned to her face and she appeared calm.

A few hours later we'd landed in Halifax and had made our way to the Casino Nova Scotia Hotel, right on the waterfront. Our room offered a great view of the waterfront, including the large and unattractive open ocean oil platform being worked on across the harbour.

Laurie went for a walk while I registered with the CISC Annual General Meeting folks and attended the National Committee on Steel Detailing Meeting. Once the meeting had concluded, I dropped off my laptop and notes in the hotel room and caught up with Laurie walking near the Bluenose II, which was stationed at Halifax during our trip. "How'd your meeting go?"

"It went fine. Are you hungry?"

"Yes," Laurie answered. "Where should we go?"

"Why don't we just grab something to eat at one of these waterfront restaurants?"

Laurie surveyed the restaurants within view. "Can we go somewhere that has something other than just seafood?"

We walked up to a restaurant that had a second floor with ample window seating that would show off the harbour. The menu had some turf items for Laurie to order and some nice surf dishes for me. There would be a slight wait for a table so we sat down on the couch in the waiting area. "Did you call home?"

"Yes," Laurie answered. "I called while you were at your meeting."

"How are the kids?"

"Ross and Eric are fine. Dana's fussing a bit about Mom giving her insulin and her blood sugar was high at snack time."

"How's your mom handling things?" I questioned.

"She's fine, I guess. I hope she can get Dana's blood sugar back down."

"Don't worry about it," I reassured her. "It sounds like everything is fine. Just enjoy yourself."

"Hey, Jim and Laurie!" Tom, a friend from another steel company, greeted us. "We've got a great table. Do you guys want to come and have dinner with Jenny and me?"

"That sounds great!" Laurie agreed.

The three of us waded through the small crowd waiting to get in and walked through to Jenny, who was already standing waiting to give Laurie and me greeting hugs. Jenny and Tom were tall and handsome athletic looking people. They have loads of energy that rubs off on you when you're with them. It was always rewarding and positive to spend some time with them.

Tom called the waiter over so that Laurie and I could order a drink and appetizer as Tom and Jenny had already ordered. "Do you know what you want for a main course?" The waiter asked me after he'd handed us two menus.

I scanned the menu quickly and decided. "I do. Are you ready Lo?"

"Yes," Laurie answered and ordered.

The waiter walked briskly to the kitchen, leaving us to talk.

"So is this your first trip without Dana?" Jenny asked Laurie.

Laurie was a bit surprised by the question, not expecting Jenny to be that up to speed with our issues. "Yes. I'm a bit nervous about it."

"Tom's told me all about it. I'd be nervous too. Have you called home already?" She asked, while Tom and I listened to the exchange.

"I called tonight, but I'm worried. This is my mom's first time looking after Dana where she has to manage everything. Dana was fussing a little bit about Mom giving her the insulin shots and her blood sugar is high."

Jenny was a good listener. She made it easy for Laurie to talk through the problems and her fears about leaving Dana for the first time since her diagnosis. Tom and I eventually tuned them out and talked about the steel fabrication industry. It wasn't long before the waiter brought the appetizers out with the drinks. His service was quick and friendly. It was my first time in Nova Scotia, but the friendliness of the people and their love of a good time shone through everywhere we went. This was a sit-down restaurant, but there was almost a pub atmosphere throughout the place that made it feel warm and inviting. I broke from the conversation, took in the atmosphere of the place for a few moments, and sipped at my Chardonnay.

"Tom, why don't we say grace and a prayer for Laurie now that our food is here?" Jenny proposed.

"That sounds fine," Tom responded.

Laurie agreed, but I didn't say anything as my mind drifted to Father Wes for a moment. Jenny and Tom held out their hands to Laurie and me so that we could form a circle with our hands around the table. Laurie and I held their hands and Jenny started into an unrehearsed grace.

"Most merciful Lord, we thank you so much for the good company that you allowed us this night. We thank you for the bountiful and nourishing food that we will enjoy in your name. We are grateful for our safe journey today and for the safe journey of our friends to Halifax. We hope that some good may come of our coming here. Also dear Lord, we offer a special prayer to you and ask that your light and goodness may shine upon Dana over these next few days while Laurie is not at home to care for her. Please guide Laurie's mom and help her to keep Dana safe and healthy. Finally Lord, please help Laurie to enjoy peace and rest while she is in Halifax. Amen."

"Very nice," Tom complimented Jenny.

"Yes, thank you very much," Laurie added.

I smiled and nodded my approval. My thoughts were conflicted. Jenny and Tom were sincere and their thoughts for us were appreciated. I could see that it made Laurie feel more welcome in this group and Jenny's show of concern seemed to lift Laurie's spirits. However, it felt awkward expressing formal reverence for God in public outside of a church. I noticed some of the people in the restaurant turn to see what we were doing while holding hands. I wondered what they thought. The potential for embarrassment left me with a self-conscious uneasiness throughout the grace and prayer.

In my mind, two thoughts pulled against each other, vying to either counter my uneasiness or strengthen its hold. I found it difficult to believe that God would listen to Jenny, no matter how sincere or caring she was. Why would God be concerned with such a small matter? However, it was impossible to ignore my hope that God would be listening. I hoped that God would not only keep Dana safe while we were here in Halifax, but that God would end her diabetes and allow her to be a normal little girl again.

While the other three continued to talk, eat, and sip at their drinks I wrestled with this issue. Even though Jenny's outward expression of love and concern made me feel awkward, deep down where my vanity could not reach, I hoped with all of my heart that her prayer was heard. I just wasn't sure.

On Thursday morning, Laurie and I decided to rent a car and drive the coastline to Lunenberg. There was a car rental agency conveniently located in the hotel and they had a mid-sized sedan available for us. It was overcast with low hanging clouds, but somehow this weather looked appropriate driving the winding roads down to Peggy's Cove. We arrived at Peggy's Cove and parked just after 10:30 am. "I'm going to go call Mom," Laurie announced. "I've got to know how the breakfast insulin went this morning."

"I'll be down by the water in front of the lighthouse."

Laurie walked into the Sou'Wester Restaurant to use the phone. I walked toward the lighthouse and the rocky shore just beyond it. If there was one place where I could count on feeling at peace it was near the ocean. I'd partially paid my way through university by becoming a scuba instructor. I forged a relationship with the ocean during those years and it had become a trusted friend that helped me to recharge my batteries whenever I neared, or better yet played deep in its embrace. The lighthouse was perched on a desolate rocky point. I found a spot to sit on the grey wave worn rocks that sloped steeply down from the lighthouse and continued down to the depths of the cold blue water. I noted the blueness of this water versus the green hue of my familiar friend, the Pacific Ocean off Vancouver Island. The swells lapped at the shore, coming close to me and then receding. I imagined what the place must be like during a real sou'wester when the monster waves would surely engulf the entire point in frothing masses of seawater. It must be breathtaking to see.

Laurie walked down the slope and sat beside me. "What's wrong?" I asked, noting the anguish on her face and the remnants of some tears.

"Dana won't take her insulin from Mom."

"What? Did she finally get her to do it?"

"Yes, but Mom's a wreck. Dana refused at first. Then, she

finally allowed Mom to do it, but moved her arm at the last second and Mom jabbed her with the needle and scratched her."

"What did she do?" I pressed.

"I was on the phone with her at that point and Mom was in tears. I told her to be forceful with Dana, to tell Dana that she was going to give her the needle and that if she pulled away again she would only get scratched again."

I put my arm around Laurie. "Did she do it?"

"Yes."

"Is she okay?"

"They'll both be fine, I guess," Laurie reasoned.

"Are you okay?"

Laurie snuggled into my shoulder and put her arm around me. "I'll be fine."

We sat for about twenty minutes just looking out into the ocean trying to forget what we couldn't. Laurie was away from Dana, but the worry was closer than ever.

"Do you want to go back to the hotel?" I finally asked.

"No," Laurie answered. "I want to see Lunenberg. There's supposed to be a great quilt shop there and I want to see it."

With that suggestion, I playfully tapped her thigh and stood up. "Let's make a move then."

Laurie stood. We walked back to the car, and continued driving down the coast toward Lunenberg. The landscape and the architecture were so much older and different than Alberta's that it was impossible not to appreciate it at least for its uniqueness. The road threaded around rocks, hills, and scenic bays revealing homes and other buildings built with styles forced upon them by the geography they inhabited. The rocks were hard and old carrying the burden of eons of erosion. The trees and vegetation staked claims to the low areas of the rocks where soil and dirt collected. Just to add even more uniqueness to the collection of eye-catching buildings was the powerful colours in which they were painted. The blues, yellows, and reds weren't pastels they were deep sky blue, lemon yellows, and fire-engine reds.

I was hungry by the time we arrived in Lunenberg, but Laurie was intent on visiting a quilt shop. We found one in the old town. The shop was an old house with low ceilings, small rooms and short doors. It had obviously stood there for some time because the floors were uneven. In fact, nothing appeared to be level anymore. It was enough to drive an engineer nuts let alone a carpenter. The air in the building was dank. It held that antique smell. Every wall in every room was covered with quilts. Some were wall hanging quilts, some were tiny, some made for king-sized beds, and they came in all kinds of colours and designs. Laurie began asking a myriad of questions of the staff so I left her and wandered from room to room looking at the selections.

I walked by the cash register and noted someone buying a quilt for $2,400! I couldn't believe what I was seeing. $2,400 for a bloody blanket! I started to look more closely at the prices on each of the quilts. It was unbelievable. I walked back to where Laurie was looking and tugged on her shoulder. "Have you seen the prices on this stuff?" I asked.

"Pretty reasonable for the work that's gone in to them, don't you think?" she answered.

"Don't get any ideas about buying one of these."

"Don't worry your head," Laurie sighed. "I'm just looking."

I heard my stomach rumble again. "When do you want to go eat?"

"I'm just about done. You can go back to the car if you want. I'll be there in a few moments."

Soon we were driving around Lunenberg searching for a good restaurant and finally settled on the Rum Runner. Once we'd finished the satisfying meal, it was time to drive back to Halifax and ready for the cocktail party at the hotel. This time we wouldn't drive the winding coastline road that took three hours from Halifax to Lunenberg. Instead, we drove the divided highway and were back in the hotel parking lot in slightly over one hour.

We dressed in formal business attire for the cocktail party, where we could mingle with leaders from the Canadian and American structural steel fabrication industry. However, the main point of the event was to hook up with some old friends and end up in a dinner party for the evening. Laurie and I were still fairly new to this crowd and it was sometimes difficult to merge into the tight social circles already developed. In the end, we enjoyed the party, met some new people, and went to dinner ourselves.

We left the hotel and took a leisurely stroll along the waterfront, holding hands, and talking. We settled on an Italian restaurant that had a quaint feel to it.

"Could I have your cell phone?" Laurie asked. "If you could get us a table, I'll call home."

"Fine," I answered and handed her the phone.

I waited in line and was seated at a great table for two near their fireplace. I ordered some appetizers and waited for Laurie to finish her phone call with Marg. She sat down at the table as the waiter brought bread. "Is everything okay?" I asked.

Laurie sighed and rubbed her forehead with her hand. "No it's not okay."

"What's wrong now?"

"Mom switched the insulin doses."

"Come-on! Poor Mom. You're kidding, right?"

"No. She gave her too much quick acting and too little long-acting. Her blood sugar is going to crash sometime tonight."

"What did you tell her to do?"

"I know I'm being overly cautious, but I'm not there," Laurie explained. "I told her she had to check Dana's blood sugar every two hours during the night. If she drops below five, I told Mom to feed her ten carbs."

"That's alright. It'll be fine. Your mom will be fine," I reassured her. "Try your best to relax."

"I can't. You know I'll never sleep tonight. I'll be thinking about this all night now. I'll be worried all weekend. I wish I was home," Laurie conceded. "I'm sorry."

CHAPTER 14

Day 4:
Saturday November 16, 2002

"Daddy, get up. Get up, Daddy," Ross begged.

I rolled over and looked at the evil alarm clock. It read 8:20 am. It was kind of weird that nobody had to get up and feed Dana before 8:00 am. I hadn't slept well last night. Nightmares came and went with regularity, knocking me from restless sleep. The different possible scenarios for Dana's coming day raced through my mind all night.

"Can I go watch TV?" Ross asked.

"No problem, pal. Wake up your little brother and let him come watch with you."

Ross hurried out of the room and let Eric, our energetic and inquisitive youngest, out of his room. I struggled out of our queen-sized bed that I had all to myself and staggered into the bathroom to shower. After cleaning up and donning some track pants and a rugby shirt, I descended the stairs, ready to give the boys some breakfast.

Sasha limped down the stairs behind me, whining the entire way. Before feeding the boys, I stuffed one of the dog's ulcer pills into her mouth. I gave her a long gentle scratch under her stomach and petted her snout. It was nice to still have her. A few weeks ago the vet thought she had cancer and wanted to do exploratory surgery. Laurie and I refused, opting for the chance that she had an ulcer. Her condition seemed to have stabilized with the pills, but she was still in some obvious discomfort.

The boys ran to the table when I called them for some hot porridge. Then the phone rang.

"Good morning," my mom Judy said.

"Hi, Mom."

"How are you doing today?" she asked.

"I'm doing fine."

"How's Dana?"

"I don't know yet. I haven't talked to Laurie this morning," I answered.

"Are you still going to bring the boys over here?"

"If it's still okay, I'd like to so that I can go to the hospital and be with Laurie and Dana."

"No problem. Just let me know when you're coming. What are you doing with Sasha?" she asked.

"Bill and Kim said they'd take her until things settle down," I responded.

"Alright. Well, call me if you need anything."

I hung up the phone, poured some cereal and milk and sat down to eat with the boys. "How'd you guys like to spend the day at Grammy's?" I asked enthusiastically.

"Oh yeah!" Ross yelled and Eric smiled at the commotion.

"Okay, let's eat breakfast, I'll call Mommy, and then we can go," I explained.

Laurie beat me to the phone call moments later.

"Hi. How was your night?" she asked, sounding tired.

"It was long. How are you?"

"I had a long night too. I forgot change for the vending machines. I was starving after you left. All of the cafeteria vendors were closed. I tried to sleep instead, but I was too hungry."

"Did you get anything to eat?" I asked.

"I went back to sit with Dana. She was sleeping so I asked one of the nurses how her blood sugar was. Of course, it was perfect because she's on an IV," Laurie jealously admitted. "Finally, one of the nurses managed to dig me up some food from the potluck the staff had."

"That was nice. Were you able to get any sleep at all?"

"I tried to, but it was impossible for a long time. There was so much spinning around in my mind."

"I know exactly how you feel."

"The only thing that allowed me to go to sleep was saying the Lord's Prayer and Hail Mary over and over until I tired."

"How's Dana today?"

"She's doing fine, I guess. The nurses woke me up after about three hours of sleep and brought me back to Dana's bed in the PICU. Dana woke up. She was hungry and thirsty and wanted to see me."

"Did you give her anything?"

"She's still not allowed to eat or drink anything," Laurie complained.

"What's on the agenda for the morning?"

"The doctors are taking her downstairs for another CAT Scan in about an hour."

"Well, I'll take the boys to Ray and Judy's and then I'll come down there to spend some time with you this afternoon. Do you need anything?"

"I don't think so."

I packed bags for Ross and Eric, found the dog's things, and loaded the truck. The boys were excited to arrive at Ray and Judy's house and ran to the front door once I'd undone their seat belts. They were there to greet them and give them hugs. Grammy's was a special place for Eric, but especially for Ross. Judy had a relationship with Ross that obliterated his apparent shyness, and replaced it with a contented, confident, beaming boy. I wished that I could bottle what she did and give Ross some of that magic wherever he went.

Ray helped me with the boys' bags and we went into the house to settle them in.

"Do you want something to eat, Jim?" Judy asked.

"I'm fine, Mom. I ate at home."

"It's no trouble you know. I could whip you up some blueberry pancakes in a jiffy."

"Leave the boy alone, Mom," Ray demanded. "He knows how to feed himself."

"Where's Dana?" Ross asked in a worried tone.

"Does he know what's going on?" Ray whispered.

I shrugged my shoulders. "I don't think he gets everything."

"Poor boy," Judy consoled. "Dana's sick and staying at the hospital with Mommy."

"I want to see her," Ross complained.

"I suppose that I could take Ross with me this afternoon, bring him back, then go back to hospital later," I reasoned. "I'll give Lo a call first to make sure she's alright with it."

I called the hospital. Dana was just about to go for her CAT scan. She remembered all of the things that she wanted now. Laurie gave me a list of clothes, books, games, videos, and dolls to bring for Dana and her for the week. She was fine with bringing Ross to the hospital to see Dana.

The boys, Grammy, and I played in the back yard for a while and Papa watched some car racing. Then we had a hearty lunch of hot soup and sandwiches.

"Okay, Grammy, Eric can go for a nap now and I'll take Rossco to see his big sister," I explained. Ross smiled, satisfied that he would soon see Dana.

"See you later, Ross," Judy waved, holding a yawning Eric to her shoulder.

Ross and I got back into the truck to drive to Sherwood Park to pick up Laurie's list of items and then go to the hospital. The cell phone rang two turns before we had reached home.

"Jim?" Laurie's controlled, but concerned voice rang out over the phone.

"Hi. What's wrong?"

"They've changed their minds. Dana's being prepped for emergency surgery right now," Laurie stated.

I slammed on the brakes of the truck without looking

behind me, veered right, and drove over the curb with the right front wheel before coming to a stop. My throat began to tighten.

"Daddy, why did you do that with the truck?" Ross yelled from the back seat.

"Just wait, Son," I scolded him. "What do you mean they're operating? The neurologist told us last night that that would be the last option. I thought they were going to let the antibiotics work?"

"The ENT came and found me after the CAT scan was finished. He'd been up all night doing Internet research on Dana's infection after arguing with the neurosurgeon against surgery."

"What did he find out?" I asked.

"He said that sometimes diabetes masks the severity of acute infections," Laurie explained. "When they looked at the CAT scan results and talked about these new findings, the team decided they had to operate on her head immediately."

Tears began to fall down my face, "What kind of operation do they need to do?"

"They showed me the CAT scan. I saw where the air bubbles are under her skull. They need to remove those. They need to remove the mastoid bone. They need to see what damage the infection has done and is doing in her head once they've opened her up to know for sure."

"How long?"

"They said it could take up to seven hours," Laurie sighed.

"Jesus Christ! They're going to open Dana's head up for seven hours?" I cried.

"Daddy, what's wrong?" Ross asked from behind.

"Just a minute, Son!"

"Are you alright, Jim?" Laurie questioned.

"No. I don't know. What am I supposed to do now?"

"I'm going down with Dana to the anesthetist in a few minutes. Once she's under, the neurologist told me that you and I should be with family to wait. I'll give them your mom and dad's number and I'll meet you there in a little while."

"Fine," my voice cracked.

"Jim. She's going to be fine. I think she's going to be fine. The doctors know what they're doing," Laurie consoled. "I'll see you in a little while. I love you."

"I love you, too."

I slowly backed the truck off the curb and drove the remainder of the way home.

"Can I still see Dana?" Ross asked, as we pulled up to the driveway.

"Not today, Son," I responded with a shaky voice. "We'll try tomorrow."

Ross looked confused and sad. I was too. Ross ran into the house upstairs to his room. I slowly exited the truck and wiped the tears from my face, allowing the weight of the situation to begin taking hold of my emotions.

"Hello, my friend," Father Wes called out as he got off his mountain bike on the driveway.

I wiped my eyes as best I could.

"Good day, Father."

"I understand there is some new trouble with little Dana," Wes said.

"More than you can believe. It's a horror story," I answered and then filled him in, stressing the gravity of the situation.

"Things will work out," Wes consoled me after hearing the story and where things stood. "Have faith in that."

"I don't have faith in that. I'm terrified I might lose my little girl. What would I do if that happened? I don't think I could recover from that."

"I understand that this is a difficult situation, but faith is what you must have now," Wes urged.

"Faith in what? I have no control over what is going to happen to my little girl. She is lying on an operating table as we speak and the surgeons are preparing to cut her head open and do God knows what to try to stop a bug that they're unsure of. I can't help her. It's ripping me up!"

Father Wes came close to me, extended his right arm, and grasped my shoulder with handshake firmness, "Listen to me carefully, Jim. I have been trying to get you to realize this for some time. Now, you must. You are a good man. Your family is a good family. But, you are alone without faith. It is wrong to be this way. Look at this situation you are in. You have done everything within your control and power to help your little girl. Have you not?"

"Of course Laurie and I have, I'd do anything to help her," I answered.

"Good. You now finally realize that it's not enough. It's never enough. Others must help, others that you can't control. Little Dana is now at the mercy of the gifts that were bestowed upon those surgeons. You can do nothing, except wait. Don't you understand how empty this situation is without faith that there is something else? Can't you see that there simply must be something else?"

"I don't know. I hope with all of my might that God is real, especially today, but I don't see it. I hope that God will help Dana, but how?"

Wes squared himself to my face and spoke once more. "God is real. You must believe it. God has a plan for everything. Have faith in that."

I shook my head and rubbed my hands rough downward over my face. "I'll try, Father."

"Now, promise me one last thing."

"What?"

"Promise me that you will pray with all of your heart for your little girl today, that your prayer will be the prayer of a man that has done all that he can to help, but needs more. Will you do that for me?" Wes urged.

"I will try my best, Father," I promised.

Wes straddled his bike and looked back at me. "Things will work out as they should, Jim. Farewell."

Father Wes eased his bike back onto the street and peddled west, away from the Alliance Church. I watched him disappear around the corner. Once Wes was gone, I did my best to gather the items that Laurie had requested. Then I entered Dana's room. I searched her room for her requested items. Dana's prized glass figurine stood on her dresser, a dolphin jumping out of the water. When show and tell time came at school, she wanted to bring this. She loved the very idea of the ocean. It drew me over and I picked up the figurine, holding it gently in my hands. Dana's room felt cold and empty, like there were no bedroom walls between me and the chill of November outside.

I knelt down at Dana's window, rested my forehead against her cold windowsill, clutching her dolphin in both hands, and closed my eyes. The emotions flooded in and out of me like a West Coast tide. I focused my mind and channeled all of my thought to Dana.

"Please God. Don't take Dana. Don't take her from this family now. We're not ready for her to go. Please leave her with us to keep this family together and strong. Please get her through this trouble and return her to health. Please give her strength to get through this fight and be a little girl again. Please let her grow up strong. I hope with all my heart that you can hear me."

"Daddy? Are you hurt, Daddy?" Ross asked from behind me.

"No, son. Daddy's fine. Do you want to go back to Grammy's now?" I answered as I staggered back to my feet, slightly embarrassed.

"Yes."

I loaded the truck with everything that we needed and retraced our route back to my childhood home in St. Albert. Judy met me at the door, gave me a hug, and began to cry. Laurie had arrived a few minutes earlier. Judy had dinner ready on the table. Eric had already eaten. Ross, Laurie, Judy, Ray, and I sat down to eat, be with each other until the hospital would call and wait for the hours to tick by.

The waiting was excruciating. The sick feeling in my stomach reminded of how I felt as Laurie was rushed into an emergency C-Section operation to give birth to Dana. Dana was in distress then and she was again, only this time the waiting was longer and my worry was worse.

"I wonder if this whole thing started with the ear infection. What if we let this happen because we didn't treat the ear infection properly?" I asked, breaking the silence of the vigil.

"Don't do that to yourself," Ray scolded me. "You didn't do this."

The phone rang. What a welcome, but terrifying sound. Laurie looked at me, let go of my hand, and picked it up.

"Hello?" she asked and then the tension drained from her face. "Hi, Mom. We're holding up. Thank you."

Marg and Norm called to give us their prayers and thoughts. Marg kept the call short knowing that we needed to keep the line clear for the hospital to call. Slowly, more calls came, and then even more. My sisters and brother called. The remainder of Laurie's family called. Uncles and aunts called. The hours began to go faster. My spirits were lifted each time I was asked to retell the stories of Dana's trials and was greeted each time with love and support. The phone rang again, and Laurie answered.

"Hello?"

There was a long pause as Laurie listened to the news. "She's out of surgery."

Our attention fixed on Laurie's every word now. She hung up. "She's out of surgery and will be in the recovery room for about an hour. Then she's going back in the PICU. She's not conscious yet," Laurie explained.

"Is she going to be okay?" I asked.

"She's fine at the moment. We can go see her now," Laurie

announced.

I got to my feet quickly, meeting Laurie's speed, and we hurried for the door.

"Good luck, you two. Don't worry about the boys," Judy encouraged.

Laurie and I took separate vehicles to the hospital because she would remain with Dana through the night. I would be returning to Judy and Ray's to sleep. We met in the parking lot and raced to the pediatric intensive care unit where Dana was being stabilized. When we arrived at the entrance to the unit, Laurie buzzed the nurse and we were allowed in. We quickly washed up and walked to Dana's bed. I was woozy, instantly. Laurie, who'd grown up in a medical family and was used to these sights, spied my oncoming condition and reached for my arm.

"Are you going to make it?" she asked.

"I'll be fine, I think. You know how I get in hospitals."

"Hang in there," she encouraged.

There were nurses and a team of doctors surrounding Dana, checking data and reading charts. We recognized most of the team by now. I didn't recognize the PICU nurses yet, but Laurie knew them from the previous night. The ENT brought us to the side and explained what they had found and what had been done to Dana. Her head was completely bandaged.

They had made a huge U-shaped incision around her left ear, starting at the base of her sideburn and ending behind and below her ear. Once they started to work on her they found extensive damage. The infection had destroyed the mastoid bone so this bone was removed. The infection had resulted in the clotting of a major draining vein in her brain, the venous sinus. Work had been done to open up this vein and remove the clot. A drill was used to bore holes through her skull to find the abscesses in her menenges in the areas of the air pockets under her skull. Once the abscess locations were discovered the infected tissue around the abscesses was cleared with a cleansing solution.

Then they looked in her left ear. The infection had destroyed the eardrum and was in the process of dislocating the tiny bones used for the majority of her hearing in the middle ear. The infection was cleared and the surgeons found a suitable piece of tissue to graft Dana a new eardrum.

"There's so much damage!" I quietly exclaimed. "What did this?"

"The lab will know in a couple of days," the ENT answered.

I walked away from the two of them and looked down at Dana. She lay motionless on the bed, in some discomfort, with tubes coming in and out in an organized chaos and white bandages covering her head. Dana's bed in the PICU was a mattress surrounded by a series of tubes with liquids and gases and intimidating equipment all around her. It looked like a lab from a science fiction horror movie. I looked around the room and was taken aback by the consistency and pace of the motion around all of the beds. I'd never been in an intensive care unit before. Someone was always moving. There was a seriousness and deliberateness to the movements. It was impossible to ignore. This was not a room designed for comfort. This was a battle zone.

I made my way back to Laurie's conversation. "Like I said, Dana will be on at least six weeks of daily intravenous antibiotic therapy and three to six months of daily injected blood thinners," the ENT explained.

"What are the blood thinners for?" I interrupted.

He looked a little annoyed at being interrupted, but held firm and professional. "They're to ensure that the work done to remove the clot in the venous sinus is successful."

"I have one more question," I announced. "Is she going to be fine?"

He thought for a moment and then answered in a sure tone. "We believe that the operation was a success. We think she's out of danger."

"Will she be able to hear in her left ear?" Laurie asked.

"We'll know fairly quickly, but I believe so," he answered.

"Did you get the bug? Can the infection come back?" I begged.

"We believe we've stopped the bug. But in truth, we won't know for sure until we monitor her for a while. We'll do another CAT scan in the morning and another MRI. She'll need to stay in PICU until mid-week and then she can most likely be moved to the regular children's ward. She'll probably stay there for a few weeks."

CHAPTER 15

Friday December 20, 2002

"Good morning Edmonton Removal Services. What news does my dad, the grim reaper bring today? Are people dying to get your business?" I greeted Ray with my too often repeated gallows humour.

Ray had worked hard his whole life to provide for his family. Fate had dealt him over a decade of particularly harsh blows in business and in his personal health. His newest venture really was grim, and definitely had zero glamour, but it provided a much needed community service. His business was basically a cadavre courier. ERS held the contract with the Capital Health Region Medical Examiner. Therefore, anytime a body needed to be transported to or from the ME, Ray's drivers completed the work. It was a brutal job, often completed under the most delicate and emotional of circumstances, such as when someone committed suicide.

I admired Ray immensely for his perseverance under difficult conditions. It would be easy for him to give up, given what he'd gone through, but he didn't. Any idiot has a chance to be successful when they actually have financial success. It takes character to amass success in the areas that really count when you don't enjoy success financially. My parents had amassed great success with friends and family, and are loved by most who know them, even though Ray's attempts to be a successful entrepreneur had not been what he'd hoped.

"I'm not actually having all that great a day," Ray answered.

"Oh. Sorry about that. What's up?" I asked, somewhat sheepishly.

"I had to make a call this morning. It was really hard. I don't think I should do calls anymore." Ray's voice began to give way from his usual on-top-of things attitude.

"Why did you have to make the call? Where are your other drivers?"

"We had a glut of out of town calls from funeral homes today, and a bunch of Medical Examiner calls. It's my first year in this business. I'd been told that Christmas time is horrible, but I had no idea that it would be this bad."

"What kind of calls are you getting?"

"People, young people with families, are taking their own lives. It's so depressing. What could go so wrong in your life that you decide to kill yourself, at Christmas?" he wondered.

"I don't know, Dad. I've never felt that way. It makes me angry when people do it, though."

"I don't understand the whole thing. Then this morning happens."

"What happened this morning?"

"I got a call from the Medical Examiner for St. Albert.

There was no one else so I took the call. When I arrived, it was horrible. It was a little boy. I don't remember how old he was. He couldn't have been eleven."

"That's terrible. What happened to him?"

"His parents brought him to the hospital with the flu last night. They went to the emergency. The doctor looked at him and sent he and his parents home with some good ideas for treating the flu."

"What? What happened to him?"

"He died four hours later!"

"My God! How?"

"They think it might have been an acute infection in the boy's head, maybe even mastoiditus," Ray explained.

"Was it strep A? That's what Dana's infection turned out to be, just regular strep throat gone nuts. Do they know what it was?"

"Not yet."

"Wow! You take it easy today. Don't push your heart too much and get a heart attack," I advised Ray.

"I'll try not to. Say, why don't you, Laurie and the kids come over for dinner tonight and keep me and Mom company?"

"That sounds fine. I'll check with Laurie, but you can expect us at about five."

After hanging up the phone with Ray, I leaned back in my chair and looked up at the ceiling in my office at Waiward. I turned the chair toward the pictures of my family that sit on top of the black cabinet. Ray's news rattled through my brain, taking my focus completely away from work. I decided to call

Laurie.

"Hello?" Laurie asked, picking up the phone in the kitchen at home.

"Hi," I answered.

"What's up, Jim?"

"Dad just called me with a story. I'm having trouble with it."

I explained Ray's story in full and Laurie listened without interruption.

"I feel absolutely horrible for those parents. I can remember exactly what it was like when I brought Dana in," Laurie sympathized.

"Wouldn't it have been excruciating? I don't want to even imagine the pain that those two must be feeling," I added.

"Oh, Jim. Remember how you've been telling me about Father Wes?"

"Of course."

"I was at my bible study course at the Alliance Church this morning. I wanted to see if I could meet him, so I asked when he would be there."

"Did you meet him?"

"No. They told me there was no Father Wes at the Alliance Church and that there never had been."

"What? Come on! Do you think I'm making this up?"

"No, but are you sure he was at the Alliance Church and not some other church?"

"Of course I'm sure!"

"Okay, okay!"

I calmed down and then remembered dinner. "Mom and

Dad invited us for dinner tonight. I told them that we'd come.
I hope that's alright?"

"That's fine. It's a little bit of a pain in the ass with all of
Dana's injections."

"Dad could use a little company tonight."

"It's fine. It's fine, I'm just complaining," Laurie conceded.

"Okay, I'll see you a little later and we'll be at Mom and
Dad's for five."

The conversations with Laurie and Ray left many questions
for me to sort through. The final hours of work ticked by
too slowly with my mind not focused on work so I asked Ted
Degner if I could leave. There was no problem with this due to
the time of year. Employees were coming and going with more
frequency anyway and it was the last Friday before most job
sites shut down for two weeks.

The first thing I wanted to find out was what happened to
Father Wes. I drove to the Alliance Church and went inside.
There was nobody to greet me at the main entrance so I
explored around a little. Finally, one of the volunteers greeted
me.

"Hello, I'm looking for one of your ministers," I greeted the
young lady.

"What's his name?"

"Father Wes."

"I don't recognize that name. Are you sure he's a minister
here?" she asked.

"Yes. I've spoken with him many times. He was here," I
answered a little brusquely.

"Alright. Let's go check with someone to find out for sure," she said, leading me to a set of offices.

We went into one of the offices and the two ladies exchanged greetings and I was then allowed to explain my question.

"I am sure that there is no Father Wes at this church," the second lady answered politely but firmly.

I rubbed my forehead a little and then asked.

"Is there anyone named Wes that is at this church?"

The lady checked her program again and then responded. "The only Wes that we've had was a janitor."

"Is he still here?"

"No. He's no longer with us."

"What was his name?"

"Wesley Pietrzyk," she answered.

"Pietrzyk? Is that Polish?" I asked.

"I don't know. I've never met the man," she admitted.

"When did he leave?" I asked.

"It says here his last shift was in the morning on November sixteenth of this year," she read. "I hope that helps you, whatever you're looking for."

I thanked the two women, left the church somewhat bewildered, and went home. Laurie was ready to go to Ray and Judy's when I arrived.

When we arrived at Ray and Judy's, Ross ran to the door. Laurie brought Eric and Dana and I brought the day bag. When our family went out to dinner you'd swear we were going on vacation. Judy opened the door and grabbed Ross. "How are you my sweet boy?" she asked him.

"I'm good."

"Do you feel better now?"

"Yes, Grammy. I'm better."

"What colour is your pee?"

"It's green again," Ross announced, to the laughter of everyone in the room.

Judy had dinner for the kids ready to go. Ross and Eric were sat at the table.

"Jim, can you do Dana's blood sugar and insulin and I'll get the plates ready?" Laurie asked.

"No problem."

"Is Ross really fine?" Judy asked, with Ray close by listening in.

"Yes he's great now. The nephrologist says his kidneys are fine and there's no noticeable blood in his urine anymore," Laurie answered for me. "We just had to monitor him for a few weeks for signs of kidney failure."

"Poor boy. With all of the horrible things happening to Dana, nobody noticed that he was really sick, too," Judy said.

"I know Mom, but surely you can understand. Besides, Rossco's as healthy as a horse. I don't think he was ever in any real trouble," I added.

"You weren't thinking that when you woke up on Sunday morning after Dana's operation and Rossco was peeing absolutely red," Ray interrupted.

"I was in no mood to mess around with my kids at that point. Laurie's brother Al thought he'd be fine, but I wanted to go to the U of A emergency anyway," I explained.

"You guys must be famous there by now," Judy said.

"You should have seen the emergency people help me that

morning. As soon as I told them who I was and what the problem was, Rossco and I were getting looked at instantly."

"It's unbelievable that Rossco had strep A attack that aggressively at the same time that Dana had it!" Ray exclaimed. "What a weekend!"

"Why did it go so differently for Ross?" Judy questioned.

"The nephrologist said that when the infection attacked Rossco, his immune system kicked into overdrive and killed it, but didn't stop there. His white blood cells were so jacked up that they started to attack his kidneys after finishing with the infection. The red pee began to flow because the filters in his kidneys were damaged allowing the blood to pass freely through."

"He didn't even complain," Judy finished. "Thank God he opened his mouth when he went to the bathroom on Sunday or we'd never have known he was really sick, too."

"Then there's Stinker Boy!" I teased Eric. "He just ate his way through all of this, smiled, and busted a few more things!"

"He's a sweet boy, too!" Judy defended Eric.

"Mom, you're so soft," I countered. "No wonder the boys love you."

I was ready with Dana's insulin after finishing her blood sugar check. I had Dana lay down on the couch and was just about to inject the insulin into her buttocks when Mom noticed.

"Why aren't you injecting into her arm or leg like you usually do?" she asked.

I finished with the injection and Dana continued with her bitter complaining about using the new site.

"Come here and have a look, Mom," I requested.

Dana protested, but I rolled up her sleeve and showed Judy the back of Dana's arms, which were hard and callused. "We can't use her leg sites right now because she gets two eighteen unit shots of her blood thinner enoxaparin every day now."

Then I pulled Dana's pants down to show Judy the Insuflon site that was subcutaneously embedded into the fat in her leg, which kept an open port for the blood thinner injections. The blood thinner bruised her leg awfully. We had to have the site switched to a different leg when the blood and bruising started to pool around her tiny knee, causing her discomfort.

"You can see now why we can't use her leg sites. The backs of her arms were the only sites we could use, but now they're so callused that the insulin doesn't get through. She doesn't have enough fat around her stomach to use that site yet, so we have to use her bum," I explained.

Ray and Judy just shook their heads in disbelief at what Dana had to endure daily.

"Mom, you should have seen some of the other kids in the Stollery. It was really humbling. I had thought we were going through hell," I commented.

"You were going through hell," Ray argued.

"The little girl next to Dana in the Stollery was having her seventeenth operation for spina bifida," Laurie commented. "That was heart breaking, but she was the sweetest kid."

"I guess we did go through hell, but we saw worse," I argued. "It could have been much worse."

The kids finished eating and started playing with some toys in the family room. The adults cleaned up, reset the table, served our food, and opened a bottle of wine. Then we sat down to eat.

"How's the dog?" Judy asked.

"She's absolutely fine. It's like nothing is wrong with her at all," Laurie answered.

"That's incredible!"

"Jim thinks it's because she was worried about Dana. I don't know," Laurie commented.

"Do you think she was giving you a signal that something was wrong?" Judy questioned.

"I don't think so," Laurie answered quickly.

"What do you think, Jim?" Ray asked.

"I don't know. Maybe."

"Laurie told me that you can't find your friend Father Wes," Judy said changing the topic.

"No. I don't know what happened there. Maybe he was just some freak janitor with a grand opinion of himself," I complained. "I hate being taken advantage of like that."

"How do you know he took advantage of you?" Ray questioned.

"I don't know that, I guess. It would have been nice if he'd said goodbye properly at least and maybe told me who he really was."

"It was terrible to hear about that little boy today, Ray. I hope you're alright," Laurie offered.

"I'll get over it. It was just a tough day. It makes you think though, doesn't it?" Ray said.

"Think about what?" I asked.

"Why did they lose their little boy and you didn't lose

Dana?" Ray asked, with his voice cracking slightly on the last word.

The four of us went silent for a long few minutes. I ate a few bites of food, sipped my wine and looked nervously at the other three.

"That's a very tough question to answer," Judy finally admitted, breaking the silence.

"What saved her?" Ray asked again. "Was it the hospital that you went to?"

"I think the U of A Hospital and especially the Stollery have some of the best medical professionals in the world. We're lucky to have them in Edmonton," Laurie reasoned.

"I agree, but the U of A normally wouldn't be your first choice for emergency would it? You live in Sherwood Park," Ray argued.

"You're right. We could have gone to the Grey Nuns in Millwoods. I've even taken the kids to St. Albert to the Sturgeon because I can get my mom to help me," Laurie admitted.

"Why did you go to the U of A?" Ray questioned.

"Dana has diabetes. Her clinic is there. I trust them," Laurie said.

"Are you suggesting that Dana wouldn't have been saved if she went to another hospital?" Judy questioned Ray.

"I don't know. My day today would certainly suggest that she'd be in a hell of lot more trouble if she wasn't at the U of A," Ray said.

"But it wasn't the diabetes that helped to diagnose the problem," I argued. "She had an ear infection. That's what drew the emergency doctor to notice the pain in her ear."

"That's right, but the boy that I picked up today only had four hours once he was brought into the hospital. Why did Dana have more time?" Ray questioned. "Isn't it because you brought her in with worsening flu symptoms that were complicating her diabetes? How long would you have waited if she wasn't diabetic?"

"I don't know," Laurie answered, thinking hard for arguments. "Maybe that played a factor."

"What did your friend Wes always want you to believe in?" Judy asked me.

"He wanted me to believe that God played a role in our lives, that God had a plan, that miracles happened," I answered.

"Maybe that's what this is then. Maybe this was a miracle," Judy suggested.

"What do you think about that?" Laurie turned and challenged me with the question she knew was toughest for me.

Judy and Ray stopped and stared at me, waiting for the answer. I poured myself another glass of wine and pondered the scope of the question. I thought about the last three years and what my family had been through, what we'd witnessed. I thought about how brave my little girl had been in facing the challenges she'd had no choice in facing and how she'd encounter so much more in her life. I thought of the things that I should face, question, and deal with. I thought about all the events, both fortunate and unfortunate, that were strung together to reach this point that I could not explain with concrete logic. I thought of how I'd been irrevocably changed.

"I don't for the life of me understand a God that can choose between that poor boy and Dana." I finally hedged.

"Yes, but was it a miracle?" all three now demanded.

"Maybe."

Laurie smiled. "Does that mean you'll come to church with me and the kids on Sunday?"

Dana and Ross ran into the room when they heard the question, with Eric toddling in behind them.

"Daddy, will you come please? And then we can go out for brunch! And then we can go swimming at Millennium Place!" Dana and Ross shouted.

"Hang on you guys! Let Daddy think," Laurie ordered. "Well Daddy, what do you think?"

I smiled, knowing defeat was imminent. "Maybe."

The kids cheered. I grabbed Dana and hugged her and Ross and Eric waited for their turn.

I wondered if there was a janitor sitting somewhere alone in the mountains by a fire, smiling, waiting for someone like me.

Hospital staff make this the best Christmas ever Daughter's life saved by skilled caring team

To the physicians, nurses and staff of the University of Alberta Hospital and the Stollery Children's Health Centre:

I am sitting in my living room with my feet up, at peace. I spent Christmas Eve at my parents' house enjoying family.

I am resting for a few hours after my family opened gifts this morning. Tonight we are going for Christmas Dinner with my wife's family.

This year I am not taking this normal agenda for granted. In fact, I can tell you all that this is without a doubt the best Christmas that I have ever had.

On November 15, 2002, the Christmas that I am now enjoying was in doubt. I was at work and my wife Laurie had just brought our Type 1 diabetic daughter Dana to emergency.

She was suffering from the flu and we had lost the battle over the last few days and nights of keeping her blood sugar levels normal and keeping her hydrated.

Within minutes after we arrived at the hospital, the emergency staff was far more interested in Dana's ear infection that was already being treated with antibiotics than they were in her flu. She, in fact, did not have the flu, and the ear infection was masking a more serious threat.

Over the next 30 hours, Dana had a large team of specialists converge on her and by late Saturday evening she'd come out of four exhausting hours of surgery on her head. She was in the hospital for close to two weeks.

It turns out that Dana's problem was a strep infection gone very nasty. It destroyed her left ear drum, mastoid bone, caused a stroke-threatening blood clot in a major vein in her head, had breached her skull, and was releasing air under her skull from abscesses near her meninges.

My wife and I were terrified at the time, and from the pace of the action around Dana we knew that she was in real danger. Even though the scope of this infection was very rare and the threat to Dana's life very real, hospital staff prevailed and even built her a new eardrum.

After the operation and all of the exhausting worrying, I began to feel sorry for Dana and for myself. How could fate deal such a blow to a little girl who'd been whacked already with diabetes?

After spending time in the Stollery Children's Health Centre with Dana over two weeks, I realized that there are many parents and children going through serious ordeals. Some situations are much more serious than ours with outcomes sure to be worse. It was humbling and eye opening.

Today, my daughter is alive, we are days away from the end of her post-operation antibiotics and blood thinner regimen, and I am going to another Christmas dinner with Laurie, Dana, Ross, and Eric. Thank you so much for that.

I hope the people who helped us have the skill, caring, and stamina to provide many, many more families with what you have given ours.

Jim Kanerva, Sherwood Park

Author's Notes:

I have done my best throughout this book to provide an experience of what life with Type 1 diabetes is like and what struggles are faced on a daily basis. However, it is hard at times to visualize what is at the working heart of this mysterious and ruinous disease. Once I'd witnessed Dana's disease for a few years, the novelty of everything new in her lifestyle was worn down. Eventually, I realized that the power of this disease, from my perspective, was its ability to pound the effectiveness of a diabetic's blood sugar management.

Imagine my little Dana, now seven years old, as born of the hardest and oldest granite on Earth from deep in the Canadian Shield. I often think of her as having granite's strength based on what she's already endured. Now imagine that there are two strong and tireless construction workers that follow her around every day and night for her entire life. The two workers each carry a five pound sledge hammer. One worker represents either a high or low blood sugar level. The other worker represents the fluctuating range in blood sugar levels.

An acceptable blood sugar level for Dana is between 5 mmol/l and 10 mmol/l. Each time Dana's blood sugar level is above 10 mmol/l or below 5 mmol/l one construction worker hammers her granite body with the sledge. Each time the range in her blood sugar level, or the difference between the highest and lowest blood sugar level of the day is above 5 mmol/l the other construction worker hammers at her granite body.

Poor blood sugar management in a Type 1 diabetic, endured over a shortened lifetime eventually results in such serious health problems as kidney failure, heart disease, impotence, blindness, amputation, and possibly death. I have provided Dana's complete January 1 – June 30, 2003 blood sugar and insulin statistics on the pages following these notes.

I invite you to analyze the results shown on the two charts and the raw data pages and imagine the hammer strokes that Dana has endured during the first six months of 2003. Think about the damage that all of these piston-like hammer strokes are causing her still developing body and mind. Realize the insidious and quiet violence that is continually pounding at her health from within. Try to visualize my wife and me experimenting, adjusting, and struggling to control blood sugar levels continually impacted by numerous internal and external factors.

I hate diabetes. It haunts my dreams for my family and for Dana.

My hope rests with God and the numerous scientists around the world that tirelessly work to find a cure. I will do what I can to help the cause.

Charts and Tables

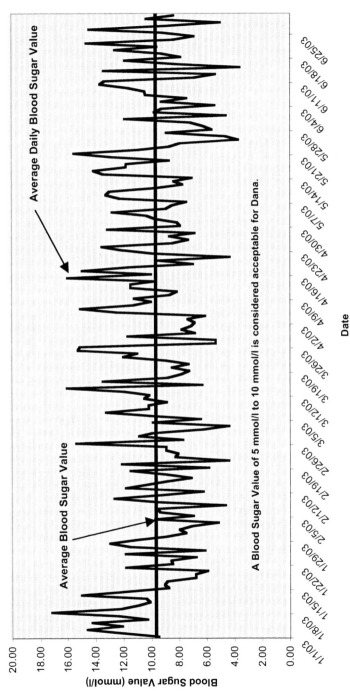

Dana's Average Daily Blood Sugar Values January 1 - June 30, 2003

Average Daily Blood Sugar Value

Average Blood Sugar Value

A Blood Sugar Value of 5 mmol/l to 10 mmol/l is considered acceptable for Dana.

Blood Sugar Value (mmol/l)

Date

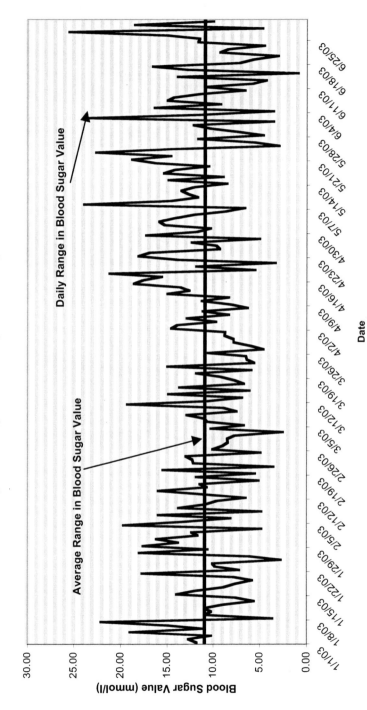

Dana's Daily Blood Sugar Value Range for January 1 - June 30, 2003

Daily Range in Blood Sugar Value

Average Range in Blood Sugar Value

Blood Sugar Value (mmol/l)

Date

Dana's Blood Sugar and Insulin Statistics for January 1 to June 30, 2003

Item	1-Jan	2-Jan	3-Jan	4-Jan	5-Jan	6-Jan	7-Jan	8-Jan	9-Jan	10-Jan	11-Jan	12-Jan	13-Jan	14-Jan	15-Jan	16-Jan	17-Jan
Breakfast Blood Sugar Value	12.7	10.7	13	5.7	16.2	19	11.3	16.6	13.9	15.5	9.1	12.4	17.6	8.2	12.6	5.8	11.2
Breakfast H Insulin	2.50	2.00	2.00	2.00	2.50	2.50	2.00	2.00	2.00	2.00	2.00	2.00	2.50	2.00	2.00	2.00	2.00
Breakfast NPH Insulin	5.00	5.00	5.00	5.00	5.00	5.50	5.00	6.00	6.00	6.00	6.00	6.00	6.00	6.00	6.50	7.00	7.00
Lunch Blood Sugar Value	9.4	12.7	9	9	8.9	4.1	4.9	15.4	12.9	15.1	8.8	12.3	12	13.5	4.3	4.6	11.3
Supper Blood Sugar Value	3.8	3.9	16.6	24.1	20	16.6	27	17.6	17.4	14.6	17.4	14.7	14.2	12.4	18.3	16.6	12.2
Supper H Insulin	0.00	0.00	0.00	0.50	0.50	0.00	0.50	0.50	1.00	0.50	0.50	0.50	0.00	0.50	1.00	1.00	1.00
Supper NPH Insulin	1.50	1.50	1.50	1.50	2.00	2.00	2.00	2.00	2.00	2.00	2.00	2.00	2.50	2.50	2.50	2.50	2.50
Night Snack Blood Sugar Value	5.8	15.2	19.2	5.1	11.7	7.4	6.6	19	6.4	7.2	6.4	5.8	16.2	15.5	6.4	9	7.1
10:00 pm to Midnight Blood Sugar Value	15.6	16.6	15.1	12.8		4.2					8.7	6.6		12.9	5.8		3.3
Midnight to 2:00 am Blood Sugar Value		13.6		15.7			12			5.3					8.1	9.2	7.9
2:00 am to 5:00 am Blood Sugar Value									10.3	7.7				7.9	5.6		
Maximum Blood Sugar Value	15.60	16.60	19.20	24.10	20.00	19.00	27.00	19.00	17.40	15.50	17.40	14.70	17.60	15.50	18.30	16.60	12.20
Minimum Blood Sugar Value	3.80	3.90	9.00	5.10	8.90	4.10	4.90	15.40	6.40	5.30	6.40	5.80	12.00	7.90	4.30	4.60	3.30
Daily Average Chart Data																	
Average Daily Blood Sugar Value	9.46	12.12	14.58	12.07	14.20	10.26	12.36	17.15	12.18	10.90	10.08	10.36	15.00	11.73	8.73	9.04	8.83
Overall Average Blood Sugar Value	9.65	9.65	9.65	9.65	9.65	9.65	9.65	9.65	9.65	9.65	9.65	9.65	9.65	9.65	9.65	9.65	9.65
Range Chart Data																	
Daily Range in Blood Sugar Values	11.80	12.70	10.20	19.00	11.10	14.90	22.10	3.60	11.00	10.20	11.00	8.90	5.60	7.60	14.00	12.00	8.90
Average Range in Blood Sugar Values	10.94	10.94	10.94	10.94	10.94	10.94	10.94	10.94	10.94	10.94	10.94	10.94	10.94	10.94	10.94	10.94	10.94

Blood Sugar Values in mmol/l and Insulin values in units (1 unit = 1/100 ml)

Dana's Blood Sugar and Insulin Statistics for January 1 to June 30, 2003

Item	18-Jan	19-Jan	20-Jan	21-Jan	22-Jan	23-Jan	24-Jan	25-Jan	26-Jan	27-Jan	28-Jan	29-Jan	30-Jan	31-Jan	1-Feb	2-Feb	3-Feb
Breakfast Blood Sugar Value	8.3	8.7	4.4	2.9	4.9	8.6	3.7	11.50	7.90	4.90	14.40	10.10	5.40	4.30	3.40	15.40	4.90
Breakfast H Insulin	2.00	2.00	2.00	2.00	2.00	1.50	1.50	1.50	2.00	2.00	2.00	2.00	2.00	1.50	1.50	1.50	1.50
Breakfast NPH Insulin	7.00	7.00	7.00	7.00	7.00	7.00	7.00	7.00	7.00	7.00	7.50	7.50	8.00	8.00	8.00	8.00	8.00
Lunch Blood Sugar Value	4.8	10.1	2.8		8.9	7.4	5.20	13.40	3.90	5.80	7.20	14.90	2.90	4.10	3.70	3.00	4.10
Supper Blood Sugar Value	11.2	5.7	6.4	13.7	6.2	15.1	13.80	10.70	9.20	22.90	17.80	20.70	12.30	3.90	15.10	3.80	8.70
Supper H Insulin	0.50	0.00	0.00	0.00	0.00	0.50	0.50	0.00	0.00	0.50	0.50	0.50	0.00	0.00	0.50	0.50	0.50
Supper NPH Insulin	2.50	2.50	2.50	2.00	2.00	2.00	2.00	2.00	2.00	2.00	2.00	2.00	2.00	2.00	1.00	1.50	1.50
Night Snack Blood Sugar Value	5.1	5.1	10.6	20.6	10.1	5.3		11.40	8.90	10.30	16.40	6.60	16.70	20.10	3.70	5.50	3.90
10:00 pm to Midnight Blood Sugar Value	7.5		5.3		12.1	7.8			3.10	13.70	9.00	10.60	10.20		13.90	7.40	4.00
Midnight to 2:00 am Blood Sugar Value	3.6			10.1		7.3	4.20	12.20					5.90	4.90			
2:00 am to 5:00 am Blood Sugar Value		4.3							3.60			3.10					
Maximum Blood Sugar Value	11.20	10.10	10.60	20.60	12.10	15.10	13.80	13.40	9.20	22.90	17.80	20.70	16.70	20.10	15.10	15.40	8.70
Minimum Blood Sugar Value	3.60	4.30	2.80	2.90	4.90	5.30	3.70	10.70	3.10	4.90	7.20	3.10	2.90	3.90	3.40	3.00	3.90
Daily Average Chart Data																	
Average Daily Blood Sugar Value	6.75	6.78	5.90	11.83	8.44	8.58	6.73	11.84	6.10	11.52	12.96	11.00	8.90	7.46	7.96	7.02	5.12
Overall Average Blood Sugar Value	9.65	9.65	9.65	9.65	9.65	9.65	9.65	9.65	9.65	9.65	9.65	9.65	9.65	9.65	9.65	9.65	9.65
Range Chart Data																	
Daily Range in Blood Sugar Values	7.60	5.80	7.80	17.70	7.20	9.80	10.10	2.70	6.10	18.00	10.60	17.60	13.80	16.20	11.70	12.40	4.80
Average Range in Blood Sugar Values	10.94	10.94	10.94	10.94	10.94	10.94	10.94	10.94	10.94	10.94	10.94	10.94	10.94	10.94	10.94	10.94	10.94

Blood Sugar Values in mmol/l and Insulin values in units (1 unit = 1/100 ml)

Dana's Blood Sugar and Insulin Statistics for January 1 to June 30, 2003

Item	4-Feb	5-Feb	6-Feb	7-Feb	8-Feb	9-Feb	10-Feb	11-Feb	12-Feb	13-Feb	14-Feb	15-Feb	16-Feb	17-Feb	18-Feb	19-Feb	20-Feb
Breakfast Blood Sugar Value	3.90	7.70	7.30	4.30	4.40	12.30	11.40	11.60	9.20	17.30	15.50	14.70	14.10	10.40	15.60	8.90	14.60
Breakfast H Insulin	1.50	1.50	1.50	1.50	1.50	1.50	1.50	1.50	1.50	1.50	1.50	1.50	1.50	1.50	1.50	1.50	1.50
Breakfast NPH Insulin	8.00	8.00	8.00	8.00	8.00	7.50	8.00	8.00	8.00	8.00	8.00	8.00	8.00	8.00	8.00	8.00	8.00
Lunch Blood Sugar Value	23.60	5.20	6.60	11.30	3.10	3.40	7.10	5.60	2.70	6.20	5.20	5.40	8.40	7.80	13.50	6.20	22.00
Supper Blood Sugar Value	4.40	3.10	14.70	10.10	5.40	17.20	16.10	15.20	6.10	14.80	19.80	12.80	4.10	7.80	3.70	5.40	8.90
Supper H Insulin	0.50	0.50	0.50	0.50	0.50	0.50	0.50	0.50	0.50	0.50	0.50	0.50	0.50	0.50	0.50	0.50	0.50
Supper NPH Insulin	1.00	1.00	1.00	1.00	1.00	1.50	1.50	1.50	1.50	1.50	1.50	1.50	1.50	1.50	1.50	2.00	2.00
Night Snack Blood Sugar Value		2.70	6.80	3.10	3.20	5.40	10.60	8.10	4.10	9.30	3.80	4.00	4.20	6.80	13.60	3.40	6.50
10.00 pm to Midnight Blood Sugar Value	7.00	15.90		19.10	3.60			7.20	8.90	11.50	7.60		6.20	11.90	11.10		8.50
Midnight to 2.00 am Blood Sugar Value			11.30		4.80		18.00	7.40				5.40	2.60			5.20	
2.00 am to 5.00 am Blood Sugar Value					7.90			9.10				11.10	9.90				
Maximum Blood Sugar Value	23.60	15.90	14.70	19.10	7.90	17.20	18.00	15.20	9.20	17.30	19.80	14.70	14.10	11.90	15.60	8.90	22.00
Minimum Blood Sugar Value	3.90	2.70	6.60	3.10	3.10	3.40	7.10	5.60	2.70	6.20	3.80	4.00	2.60	6.80	3.70	3.40	6.50
Daily Average Chart Data																	
Average Daily Blood Sugar Value	9.73	6.92	9.34	9.58	4.63	9.58	12.64	9.17	6.20	11.82	10.38	8.90	7.07	8.94	11.50	5.82	12.10
Overall Average Blood Sugar Value	9.65	9.65	9.65	9.65	9.65	9.65	9.65	9.65	9.65	9.65	9.65	9.65	9.65	9.65	9.65	9.65	9.65
Range Chart Data																	
Daily Range in Blood Sugar Values	19.70	13.20	8.10	16.00	4.80	13.80	10.90	9.60	6.50	11.10	16.00	10.70	11.50	5.10	11.90	5.50	15.50
Average Range in Blood Sugar Values	10.94	10.94	10.94	10.94	10.94	10.94	10.94	10.94	10.94	10.94	10.94	10.94	10.94	10.94	10.94	10.94	10.94

Blood Sugar Values in mmol/l and Insulin values in units (1 unit = 1/100 ml)

Dana's Blood Sugar and Insulin Statistics for January 1 to June 30, 2003

Item	21-Feb	22-Feb	23-Feb	24-Feb	25-Feb	26-Feb	27-Feb	28-Feb	1-Mar	2-Mar	3-Mar	4-Mar	5-Mar	6-Mar	7-Mar	8-Mar	9-Mar
Breakfast Blood Sugar Value	6.10	16.10	4.90	16.70	11.00	16.20	12.80	13.70	14.70	5.80	4.60	9.30	4.30	13.30	18.40	7.00	11.10
Breakfast H Insulin	1.50	1.50	1.50	2.50	2.00	2.00	2.00	2.00	2.00	2.00	2.00	2.00	2.00	2.00	2.50	2.00	2.00
Breakfast NPH Insulin	8.00	8.00	8.00	7.00	7.00	7.00	7.00	7.00	7.00	7.00	7.00	7.00	7.00	7.00	7.00	7.00	7.00
Lunch Blood Sugar Value	2.60	4.90	5.30	6.80	7.80	16.40	12.90	8.80	6.20	3.80	5.00	9.70	5.70	8.10	7.40	16.90	14.20
Supper Blood Sugar Value	4.80	10.40	3.70	8.10	11.60	19.10	3.90	14.60	6.30	7.90	5.40		3.40	3.70	13.80	15.10	12.90
Supper H Insulin	0.50	0.50	0.00	0.50	0.50	0.50	0.50	0.50	0.00	0.00	0.00	0.00	0.00	0.00	0.00	0.50	0.50
Supper NPH Insulin	2.00	2.00	0.00	1.00	1.00	1.50	1.50	1.50	2.00	2.00	2.00	2.00	2.00	1.50	2.00	1.50	1.50
Night Snack Blood Sugar Value	4.10	8.70	10.30	3.70	7.40	16.20	4.00	11.10	14.00	10.80	5.40	15.40	10.10	10.40	18.20	4.00	8.20
10:00 pm to Midnight Blood Sugar Value	3.70	5.60	16.00	9.30	6.70		4.40	6.20		3.10	2.90					7.70	6.70
Midnight to 2:00 am Blood Sugar Value	4.90	3.90					4.80		8.10		3.90	5.10	6.40	14.40	8.40		8.00
2:00 am to 5:00 am Blood Sugar Value						9.00	11.10				3.30		8.40				
Maximum Blood Sugar Value	6.10	16.10	16.00	16.70	11.60	19.10	12.90	14.60	14.70	10.80	5.40	15.40	10.10	14.40	18.40	16.90	14.20
Minimum Blood Sugar Value	2.60	3.90	3.70	3.70	6.70	9.00	3.90	6.20	6.20	3.10	2.90	5.10	3.40	3.70	7.40	4.00	6.70
Daily Average Chart Data																	
Average Daily Blood Sugar Value	4.37	8.27	8.04	8.92	8.90	15.38	7.70	10.88	9.86	6.28	4.36	9.88	6.38	9.98	13.24	10.14	10.18
Overall Average Blood Sugar Value	9.65	9.65	9.65	9.65	9.65	9.65	9.65	9.65	9.65	9.65	9.65	9.65	9.65	9.65	9.65	9.65	9.65
Range Chart Data																	
Daily Range in Blood Sugar Values	3.50	12.20	12.30	13.00	4.90	10.10	9.00	8.40	8.50	7.70	2.50	10.30	6.70	10.70	11.00	12.90	7.50
Average Range in Blood Sugar Values	10.94	10.94	10.94	10.94	10.94	10.94	10.94	10.94	10.94	10.94	10.94	10.94	10.94	10.94	10.94	10.94	10.94

Blood Sugar Values in mmol/l and Insulin values in units (1 unit = 1/100 ml)

Dana's Blood Sugar and Insulin Statistics for January 1 to June 30, 2003

Item	10-Mar	11-Mar	12-Mar	13-Mar	14-Mar	15-Mar	16-Mar	17-Mar	18-Mar	19-Mar	20-Mar	21-Mar	22-Mar	23-Mar	24-Mar	25-Mar	26-Mar
Breakfast Blood Sugar Value	12.10	22.40	10.40	16.30	17.60	6.80	12.20	13.10	6.40	7.20	15.40	9.20	19.30	10.10	10.70	17.90	16.60
Breakfast H Insulin	2.00	2.00	2.00	2.50	2.00	2.00	2.00	2.00	2.00	2.00	2.00	2.00	2.00	2.00	2.00	2.50	2.50
Breakfast NPH Insulin	7.00	7.00	7.00	7.00	7.00	7.00	7.00	7.00	7.00	7.00	7.00	7.00	7.00	7.00	7.00	7.00	7.00
Lunch Blood Sugar Value	6.20	21.30	8.90	9.80	15.90	3.60	6.60	7.70	11.60	12.40	5.10	3.30	5.80	9.40	11.10	11.40	14.60
Supper Blood Sugar Value	3.70	8.20	3.60	9.40	25.20	4.40	12.50	8.90	8.10	3.30	7.60	8.00	4.30	15.00	7.70	17.60	9.30
Supper H Insulin	0.50	0.00	0.00	0.00	0.50	0.00	0.00	0.00	0.00	0.00	0.00	0.00	0.00	0.00	0.00	0.50	0.50
Supper NPH Insulin	1.50	2.00	1.50	2.00	1.50	2.00	2.00	2.00	2.00	2.00	1.50	1.50	1.50	1.50	1.50	1.50	1.50
Night Snack Blood Sugar Value	9.70	10.20	14.30	9.50	10.30	9.70	20.30	6.40	9.40	9.30	3.50	7.20	8.80	11.80	11.60	14.10	19.90
10:00 pm to Midnight Blood Sugar Value	12.60	3.10	10.80	14.80	11.20		15.70	8.00		8.00	10.90	7.10		13.70	10.70		
Midnight to 2:00 am Blood Sugar Value		5.10	12.70			4.60			3.90			8.80	6.60		14.10		
2:00 am to 5:00 am Blood Sugar Value		3.20				8.50			7.60	3.20							
Maximum Blood Sugar Value	12.60	22.40	14.30	16.30	25.20	9.70	20.30	13.10	11.60	12.40	15.40	9.20	19.30	15.00	14.10	17.90	19.90
Minimum Blood Sugar Value	3.70	3.10	3.60	9.40	10.30	3.60	6.60	6.40	3.90	3.20	3.50	3.30	4.30	9.40	7.70	11.40	9.30
Daily Average Chart Data																	
Average Daily Blood Sugar Value	8.86	10.50	10.12	11.96	16.04	6.27	13.46	8.82	7.83	7.23	8.50	7.27	8.96	12.00	10.98	15.25	15.10
Overall Average Blood Sugar Value	9.65	9.65	9.65	9.65	9.65	9.65	9.65	9.65	9.65	9.65	9.65	9.65	9.65	9.65	9.65	9.65	9.65
Range Chart Data																	
Daily Range in Blood Sugar Values	8.90	19.30	10.70	6.90	14.90	6.10	13.70	6.70	7.70	9.20	11.90	5.90	15.00	5.60	6.40	6.50	10.60
Average Range in Blood Sugar Values	10.94	10.94	10.94	10.94	10.94	10.94	10.94	10.94	10.94	10.94	10.94	10.94	10.94	10.94	10.94	10.94	10.94

Blood Sugar Values in mmol/l and Insulin values in units (1 unit = 1/100 ml)

Dana's Blood Sugar and Insulin Statistics for January 1 to June 30, 2003

Item	27-Mar	28-Mar	29-Mar	30-Mar	31-Mar	1-Apr	2-Apr	3-Apr	4-Apr	5-Apr	6-Apr	7-Apr	8-Apr	9-Apr	10-Apr	11-Apr	12-Apr
Breakfast Blood Sugar Value	5.30	9.70	16.10	4.70	12.60	11.10	17.90	17.30	4.50	14.40	17.30	13.80	12.10	7.50	14.80	8.10	21.10
Breakfast H Insulin	2.00	2.00	2.00	2.00	2.00	2.00	2.00	2.00	1.50	1.50	1.50	1.50	1.50	1.50	2.00	2.00	2.00
Breakfast NPH Insulin	7.00	7.00	7.00	7.00	7.00	7.00	7.00	6.00	6.00	6.00	6.00	6.00	6.00	6.00	6.00	6.00	6.00
Lunch Blood Sugar Value	8.00	5.30	8.30	8.30	5.70	4.20	4.10	3.40	3.10	11.00	14.90	17.50	8.70	10.20	12.80	4.60	9.80
Supper Blood Sugar Value	3.40	3.70	10.20	4.60	3.80	10.80	4.30	5.90	4.20	3.70	11.60	9.10	13.80	15.60	7.80	3.70	
Supper H Insulin	0.00	0.00	0.00	0.00	0.00	0.00	0.00	0.00	0.00	0.00	0.00	0.50	0.50	0.50	0.50	0.50	0.50
Supper NPH Insulin	2.00	2.00	2.00	1.00	1.50	1.50	1.50	1.50	1.50	1.50	1.50	1.50	1.50	1.50	1.50	1.50	1.50
Night Snack Blood Sugar Value	4.40	4.00	15.10	6.70	8.40	2.40	4.10	4.70	5.80	16.60	19.90	6.30	7.90	14.70	3.50	9.60	8.90
10:00 pm to Midnight Blood Sugar Value	3.40	3.90	8.70	4.60	8.50	3.90	3.30	6.60	12.80	16.60		9.60	7.50	8.10		10.80	6.10
Midnight to 2:00 am Blood Sugar Value		5.40		6.40		10.20	7.30				11.70				4.90	12.00	
2:00 am to 5:00 am Blood Sugar Value	7.50			12.40				6.30							8.20		
Maximum Blood Sugar Value	8.00	9.70	16.10	12.40	12.60	11.10	17.90	17.30	12.80	16.60	19.90	17.50	13.80	15.60	14.80	12.00	21.10
Minimum Blood Sugar Value	3.40	3.70	8.30	4.60	3.80	2.40	3.30	3.40	3.10	3.70	11.60	6.30	7.50	7.50	3.50	3.70	6.10
Daily Average Chart Data																	
Average Daily Blood Sugar Value	5.33	5.33	11.68	6.81	7.80	7.10	6.83	7.37	6.08	12.46	15.08	11.26	10.00	11.22	8.67	8.13	11.48
Overall Average Blood Sugar Value	9.65	9.65	9.65	9.65	9.65	9.65	9.65	9.65	9.65	9.65	9.65	9.65	9.65	9.65	9.65	9.65	9.65
Range Chart Data																	
Daily Range in Blood Sugar Values	4.60	6.00	7.80	7.80	8.80	8.70	14.60	13.90	9.70	12.90	8.30	11.20	6.30	8.10	11.30	8.30	15.00
Average Range in Blood Sugar Values	10.94	10.94	10.94	10.94	10.94	10.94	10.94	10.94	10.94	10.94	10.94	10.94	10.94	10.94	10.94	10.94	10.94

Blood Sugar Values in mmol/l and Insulin values in units (1 unit = 1/100 ml)

Dana's Blood Sugar and Insulin Statistics for January 1 to June 30, 2003

Item	13-Apr	14-Apr	15-Apr	16-Apr	17-Apr	18-Apr	19-Apr	20-Apr	21-Apr	22-Apr	23-Apr	24-Apr	25-Apr	26-Apr	27-Apr	28-Apr	29-Apr
Breakfast Blood Sugar Value	6.30	10.90	23.60	21.20	21.40	14.60	8.60	4.60	3.40	8.40	21.60	16.00	11.40	13.60	8.40	7.40	20.40
Breakfast H Insulin	2.00	2.00	2.00	2.00	2.00	2.50	2.00	2.00	2.00	2.00	2.50	2.00	2.00	2.00	2.00	2.00	2.50
Breakfast NPH Insulin	6.00	6.00	6.00	6.50	6.50	6.50	6.50	6.50	6.50	6.50	6.00	6.50	6.50	6.50	6.50	6.50	6.50
Lunch Blood Sugar Value	9.80	7.20	13.80	16.40	12.80	24.40	4.40	4.40	4.10	3.90	11.40	12.60	12.20	6.40	6.20	4.30	10.00
Supper Blood Sugar Value	18.90	9.80	20.00	3.90	5.80	3.20	9.10	11.70	3.60	5.70	3.50	24.60	10.70	6.10	3.20	9.30	3.10
Supper H Insulin	0.50	0.50	0.50	0.00	0.00	0.00	0.00	0.00	0.00	0.00	0.00	0.50	0.00	0.00	0.00	0.00	0.00
Supper NPH Insulin	1.50	1.50	1.50	1.50	2.00	2.00	2.00	2.00	2.00	2.00	2.00	2.00	2.00	2.00	2.00	2.00	2.00
Night Snack Blood Sugar Value	8.80	4.10	5.00	3.60	20.90	11.70	7.10	16.30	6.70	13.60	12.90	12.20	9.30	10.60	15.60	4.30	18.30
10:00 pm to Midnight Blood Sugar Value	13.60	8.30	17.60	6.90		4.20		10.30	3.80	17.80	9.40	8.00	2.90	3.90	10.00	8.80	
Midnight to 2:00 am Blood Sugar Value				8.00			3.60				14.20	7.70	5.00	5.60			13.80
2:00 am to 5:00 am Blood Sugar Value		17.70			13.80		8.90						7.90	4.90			
Maximum Blood Sugar Value	18.90	17.70	23.60	21.20	21.40	24.40	9.10	16.30	6.70	17.80	21.60	24.60	12.20	13.60	15.60	9.30	20.40
Minimum Blood Sugar Value	6.30	4.10	5.00	3.60	5.80	3.20	3.60	4.40	3.40	3.90	3.50	7.70	2.90	3.90	3.20	4.30	3.10
Daily Average Chart Data																	
Average Daily Blood Sugar Value	11.48	9.67	16.00	10.00	14.94	11.62	6.95	9.46	4.32	9.88	12.17	13.52	8.49	7.30	8.68	6.82	13.12
Overall Average Blood Sugar Value	9.65	9.65	9.65	9.65	9.65	9.65	9.65	9.65	9.65	9.65	9.65	9.65	9.65	9.65	9.65	9.65	9.65
Range Chart Data																	
Daily Range in Blood Sugar Values	12.60	13.60	18.60	17.60	15.60	21.20	5.50	11.90	3.30	13.90	18.10	16.90	9.30	9.70	12.40	5.00	17.30
Average Range in Blood Sugar Values	10.94	10.94	10.94	10.94	10.94	10.94	10.94	10.94	10.94	10.94	10.94	10.94	10.94	10.94	10.94	10.94	10.94

Blood Sugar Values in mmol/l and Insulin values in units (1 unit = 1/100 ml)

Dana's Blood Sugar and Insulin Statistics for January 1 to June 30, 2003

Item	30-Apr	1-May	2-May	3-May	4-May	5-May	6-May	7-May	8-May	9-May	10-May	11-May	12-May	13-May	14-May	15-May	16-May
Breakfast Blood Sugar Value	15.10	11.90	13.70	9.80	17.10	16.00	13.00	11.30	10.60	19.50	19.10	17.10	5.50	16.70	11.90	17.10	19.80
Breakfast H Insulin	2.00	2.00	2.00	2.00	2.50	2.00	2.50	2.50	0.00	2.50	3.00	3.00	2.50	2.50	2.50	2.50	2.50
Breakfast NPH Insulin	6.50	6.50	6.50	6.50	6.50	6.50	6.50	6.50	0.00	6.50	6.50	6.50	6.50	6.50	6.50	6.50	6.50
Lunch Blood Sugar Value	9.20	2.90	18.30	2.80	17.20	5.80	4.30	4.70	27.80	15.10	9.60	8.50	4.70	4.60	10.40	15.20	10.90
Supper Blood Sugar Value	3.30	4.40	3.90	4.60	15.50	14.70	4.60	8.90	13.70	14.20	15.10	12.40	6.90	10.20	3.40	12.90	12.40
Supper H Insulin	0.00	0.00	0.00	0.00	0.50	0.50	0.00	0.00	0.50	0.50	0.50	0.50	0.50	0.50	0.50	0.50	0.50
Supper NPH Insulin	2.00	2.00	2.00	2.00	2.00	1.50	2.00	2.00	1.50	2.00	2.00	2.00	2.00	2.00	2.00	2.00	2.00
Night Snack Blood Sugar Value	4.70	5.70	11.50	18.70	11.20	3.90	9.60	5.50	3.90	17.00	7.40	4.40	4.20	6.50	4.70	20.50	15.20
10:00 pm to Midnight Blood Sugar Value	7.20	10.70	3.00		3.00	4.30	10.90	6.60	8.10	8.70	13.70	6.80	7.30	6.80	4.70	5.60	12.30
Midnight to 2:00 am Blood Sugar Value			7.90	15.70					9.30	4.90		8.80	17.70	5.50		9.20	
2:00 am to 5:00 am Blood Sugar Value		13.20						7.50									
Maximum Blood Sugar Value	15.10	13.20	18.30	18.70	17.20	16.00	13.00	11.30	27.80	19.50	19.10	17.10	17.70	16.70	11.90	20.50	19.80
Minimum Blood Sugar Value	3.30	2.90	3.00	2.80	3.00	3.90	4.30	4.70	3.90	4.90	7.40	4.40	4.20	4.60	3.40	5.60	10.90
Daily Average Chart Data																	
Average Daily Blood Sugar Value	7.90	8.13	9.72	10.32	12.80	8.94	8.48	7.42	12.23	13.23	12.98	9.67	7.72	8.38	7.02	13.42	14.12
Overall Average Blood Sugar Value	9.65	9.65	9.65	9.65	9.65	9.65	9.65	9.65	9.65	9.65	9.65	9.65	9.65	9.65	9.65	9.65	9.65
Range Chart Data																	
Daily Range in Blood Sugar Values	11.80	10.30	15.30	15.90	14.20	12.10	8.70	6.60	23.90	14.60	11.70	12.70	13.50	12.10	8.50	14.90	8.90
Average Range in Blood Sugar Values	10.94	10.94	10.94	10.94	10.94	10.94	10.94	10.94	10.94	10.94	10.94	10.94	10.94	10.94	10.94	10.94	10.94

Blood Sugar Values in mmol/l and Insulin values in units (1 unit = 1/100 ml)

Dana's Blood Sugar and Insulin Statistics for January 1 to June 30, 2003

Item	17-May	18-May	19-May	20-May	21-May	22-May	23-May	24-May	25-May	26-May	27-May	28-May	29-May	30-May	31-May	1-Jun	2-Jun
Breakfast Blood Sugar Value	18.30	18.70	8.70	18.00	14.10	18.40	25.30	17.60	5.80	8.50	15.50	8.30	10.70	9.40	16.40	5.10	5.50
Breakfast H Insulin	4.00	3.00	3.00	3.50	4.50	4.00	4.00	3.50	3.00	3.00	3.00	3.00	3.00	3.00	3.00	3.00	2.50
Breakfast NPH Insulin	7.00	6.50	6.50	7.50	7.00	8.00	8.00	7.00	7.00	6.50	6.50	6.50	6.50	6.50	6.50	6.50	6.00
Lunch Blood Sugar Value	20.60	13.20	12.80	19.80	27.00	3.80	6.20		3.70	2.90	4.00	3.80	6.60	2.70	4.20	3.40	27.80
Supper Blood Sugar Value	8.90	17.70	3.40	3.50	20.00	11.50	2.70	3.50	3.10	3.40	3.80	3.70	3.30	4.60	9.90	4.10	6.50
Supper H Insulin	1.00	1.00	0.50	0.50	1.00	0.50	0.50	0.50	0.50	0.50	0.00	0.00	0.00	0.00	0.00	0.00	0.00
Supper NPH Insulin	2.00	2.00	2.00	2.50	2.50	3.50	3.50	3.00	2.50	2.00	2.50	2.50	2.50	2.50	2.50	2.50	2.00
Night Snack Blood Sugar Value	5.20	16.00	6.10	16.90	8.30	5.70	3.60	3.60	3.10	3.80	13.20	7.00	6.90	3.80	14.70	5.20	4.20
10:00 pm to Midnight Blood Sugar Value	7.20	7.70	7.20	6.20	8.20	15.30		4.60	2.90	4.60	8.00	5.20			15.80	3.10	4.80
Midnight to 2:00 am Blood Sugar Value	10.60	4.60	13.90				4.80	3.00	3.60				3.70	9.30	15.40		
2:00 am to 5:00 am Blood Sugar Value		4.50					9.60	15.00						13.00	6.80	6.60	
Maximum Blood Sugar Value	20.60	18.70	13.90	19.80	27.00	18.40	25.30	17.60	5.80	8.50	15.50	8.30	10.70	13.00	16.40	6.60	27.80
Minimum Blood Sugar Value	5.20	4.50	3.40	3.50	8.20	3.80	2.70	3.00	2.90	2.90	3.80	3.70	3.30	2.70	4.20	3.10	4.20
Daily Average Chart Data																	
Average Daily Blood Sugar Value	11.80	11.77	8.68	12.88	15.52	10.94	8.70	7.88	3.70	4.64	8.90	5.60	6.24	7.13	11.89	4.58	9.76
Overall Average Blood Sugar Value	9.65	9.65	9.65	9.65	9.65	9.65	9.65	9.65	9.65	9.65	9.65	9.65	9.65	9.65	9.65	9.65	9.65
Range Chart Data																	
Daily Range in Blood Sugar Values	15.40	14.20	10.50	16.30	18.80	14.60	22.60	14.60	2.90	5.60	11.70	4.60	7.40	10.30	12.20	3.50	23.60
Average Range in Blood Sugar Values	10.94	10.94	10.94	10.94	10.94	10.94	10.94	10.94	10.94	10.94	10.94	10.94	10.94	10.94	10.94	10.94	10.94

Blood Sugar Values in mmol/l and Insulin values in units (1 unit = 1/100 ml)

Dana's Blood Sugar and Insulin Statistics for January 1 to June 30, 2003

Item	3-Jun	4-Jun	5-Jun	6-Jun	7-Jun	8-Jun	9-Jun	10-Jun	11-Jun	12-Jun	13-Jun	14-Jun	15-Jun	16-Jun	17-Jun	18-Jun	19-Jun
Breakfast Blood Sugar Value	6.20	7.40	5.70	9.70	17.80	18.20	19.10	10.70	17.70	9.80	4.90	14.80	3.40	10.90	16.70	8.80	12.00
Breakfast H Insulin	2.00	2.00	2.00	2.00	2.50	3.00	3.00	2.50	3.00	3.00	2.50	2.50	2.50	2.50	2.50	2.50	2.50
Breakfast NPH Insulin	5.00	5.00	5.00	5.00	5.00	5.00	5.00	5.00	5.50	5.50	5.50	5.50	5.50	5.50	5.50	5.50	5.50
Lunch Blood Sugar Value	8.30	5.00	2.40	3.20	13.40	14.10	14.90	13.70	18.10	7.40	4.50	6.80	3.20	1.90	7.30	10.90	6.30
Supper Blood Sugar Value	9.30	4.60	7.30	12.40	6.30	10.70	9.00	17.30	10.40	4.00	3.80	6.20	3.60	7.80	9.40	8.80	7.40
Supper H Insulin	0.00	0.00	0.00	0.50	0.00	0.00	0.00	0.50	0.50	0.00	0.00	0.00	0.00	0.00	0.00	0.00	0.00
Supper NPH Insulin	2.50	2.50	2.50	2.50	2.50	2.50	2.50	2.50	2.50	3.00	3.00	3.00	3.00	3.00	3.00	3.00	3.00
Night Snack Blood Sugar Value	16.90	3.90	18.80	8.00	2.80	5.40	10.30	12.40	7.10	6.30	6.60	20.10	4.10	14.70	21.30	8.50	11.40
10:00 pm to Midnight Blood Sugar Value	5.40	7.40	12.10	3.70	8.40	3.90		13.10	13.30			16.60	3.60	5.90		6.40	9.30
Midnight to 2:00 am Blood Sugar Value		4.00					7.70				8.10	15.90			4.70	3.70	
2:00 am to 5:00 am Blood Sugar Value					13.60		9.30	14.70			4.20						
Maximum Blood Sugar Value	16.90	7.40	18.80	12.40	17.80	18.20	19.10	17.30	18.10	9.80	8.10	20.10	4.10	14.70	21.30	10.90	12.00
Minimum Blood Sugar Value	5.40	3.90	2.40	3.20	2.80	3.90	7.70	10.70	7.10	4.00	3.80	6.20	3.20	1.90	4.70	3.70	6.30
Daily Average Chart Data																	
Average Daily Blood Sugar Value	9.22	5.38	9.26	7.40	10.38	10.46	11.72	13.65	13.32	6.88	5.35	13.40	3.58	8.24	11.88	7.85	9.28
Overall Average Blood Sugar Value	9.65	9.65	9.65	9.65	9.65	9.65	9.65	9.65	9.65	9.65	9.65	9.65	9.65	9.65	9.65	9.65	9.65
Range Chart Data																	
Daily Range in Blood Sugar Values	11.50	3.50	16.40	9.20	15.00	14.30	11.40	6.60	11.00	5.80	4.30	13.90	0.90	12.80	16.60	7.20	5.70
Average Range in Blood Sugar Values	10.94	10.94	10.94	10.94	10.94	10.94	10.94	10.94	10.94	10.94	10.94	10.94	10.94	10.94	10.94	10.94	10.94

Blood Sugar Values in mmol/l and Insulin values in units (1 unit = 1/100 ml)

Dana's Blood Sugar and Insulin Statistics for January 1 to June 30, 2003

Item	20-Jun	21-Jun	22-Jun	23-Jun	24-Jun	25-Jun	26-Jun	27-Jun	28-Jun	29-Jun	30-Jun	Averages
Breakfast Blood Sugar Value	10.70	4.30	14.90	7.60	15.20	4.80	8.80	7.60	4.90	4.80	12.70	11.70
Breakfast H Insulin	2.50	2.50	2.50	2.50	2.50	2.50	2.50	2.00	2.50	2.50	2.50	2.16
Breakfast NPH Insulin	5.50	5.50	5.50	6.00	5.50	5.50	5.50	5.00	5.50	5.50	5.00	6.56
Lunch Blood Sugar Value		8.70	14.80	10.90	5.70	9.70	6.30	27.80	8.10	8.50	8.90	9.05
Supper Blood Sugar Value		9.30	19.00	10.20	6.10	11.20	21.30	2.30	4.10	2.80	10.90	9.63
Supper H Insulin	0.00	0.00	0.50	0.00	0.00	0.00	0.00	0.00	0.00	0.00	0.00	0.26
Supper NPH Insulin	3.00	3.00	3.00	3.00	3.00	3.00	3.00	3.00	3.00	3.00	3.00	2.00
Night Snack Blood Sugar Value	13.40	13.60	10.60	6.90	7.20	16.30	18.40		6.10	21.30	10.40	9.45
10:00 pm to Midnight Blood Sugar Value	13.70	11.90	13.80	6.40	3.50	6.00	17.40	3.00	3.40	13.80	6.80	8.52
Midnight to 2:00 am Blood Sugar Value					4.70	7.10		4.30	3.40		2.70	7.81
2:00 am to 5:00 am Blood Sugar Value					5.70					10.80	6.10	8.52
Maximum Blood Sugar Value	13.70	13.60	19.00	10.90	15.20	16.30	21.30	27.80	8.10	21.30	12.70	11.70
Minimum Blood Sugar Value	10.70	4.30	10.60	6.40	3.50	4.80	6.30	2.30	3.40	2.80	2.70	7.81
Daily Average Chart Data												
Average Daily Blood Sugar Value	12.60	9.56	14.62	8.40	6.87	9.18	14.44	9.00	5.00	10.33	8.36	9.65
Overall Average Blood Sugar Value	9.65	9.65	9.65	9.65	9.65	9.65	9.65	9.65	9.65	9.65	9.65	9.65
Range Chart Data												
Daily Range in Blood Sugar Values	3.00	9.30	8.40	4.50	11.70	11.50	15.00	25.50	4.70	18.50	10.00	10.94
Average Range in Blood Sugar Values	10.94	10.94	10.94	10.94	10.94	10.94	10.94	10.94	10.94	10.94	10.94	10.94

Blood Sugar Values in mmol/l and Insulin values in units (1 unit = 1/100 ml)

ISBN 1-41204347-6